MOST OF
MY PATIENTS
ARE ANIMALS

MOST OF
MY PATIENTS
ARE ANIMALS

Robert M. Miller

With an Introduction by
James Herriot

A STAR BOOK
published by
the Paperback Division of
W H Allen & Co Plc

A Star Book
Published in 1988
by the Paperback Division of
W H Allen & Co Plc
44 Hill Street
London W1X 8LB

First published in Great Britain by
W H Allen & Co Plc, 1987

Printed and bound in Great Britain by
Anchor Brendon Ltd, Tiptree, Essex

ISBN 0 352 32089 3

Grateful acknowledgment is made to the Veterinary
Publishing Company of Edwardsville, Kansas, for
permission to use material published by them; the
author also wishes to express his appreciation to
American Veterinary Publications, Inc. of Santa
Barbara, California, for granting permission to
reprint cartoons from the RMM books, *Who Has
the 9:30 Appointment* and *RMM Strikes Again*.

To Mark and Laurel, with love

Introduction

by

James Herriot

Some ten years ago I was sitting in solitary state in my kitchen in Yorkshire, drinking my morning cup of tea and allowing the world to creep up on me. At the same time I was opening my mail and was totally unprepared for a letter from America which began, 'Dear Sir, You are a scoundrel. You have plagiarized my entire life.' I almost spilled my tea, and as I read on found I was being accused of a wide variety of misrepresentations. 'The setting of your book was not the Yorkshire dales and moors, it was the mountains and valleys of southwestern Montana. And when you describe how you had to climb through the ceiling to escape from a kicking cow, that was on the Parini place, just a few miles east of here, I remember it too well.' I had begun to tremble, and it was not until the writer exploded, 'Anyway, your wife's name is not Helen, it's Dorothy!' that I realized I was having my leg pulled.

The nice man who wrote was an eminent American veterinarian named Harry Furgeson, and it was his humorous way of expressing a fact that is so very true – that the things that have happened to me have happened to fellow veterinarians all over the world.

This has been the source of many happy meetings with my colleagues in other countries. We have swapped experiences, listened to the successes and failures that are part of the veterinary life, and shared congratulations and commiserations. Most of all, we have laughed together, because the life of the veterinarian is spiced with laughter. Animals are unpredictable things, and when they are sick, anything

7

can happen. And whereas a physician's human patients are usually trying to cooperate with him, ours are invariably trying to thwart us at every turn. This state of affairs gives rise to situations that can be embarrassing, humiliating, dangerous, and occasionally terrifying. However, these things, though traumatic at the time, are often funny in retrospect, and it was this aspect of my professional life that motivated me to start writing in the first place. Veterinary practice, of course, has its sad side. Animals are totally vulnerable: they are dependent on us, and it is unforgiveable to let them down. I think it is this fact that engenders the deep pull that they have on our emotions.

Working with animals, despite the regular contretemps, adds up to a rewarding and fulfilling life, which is confirmed by the fact that most vets seem to be happy men. They are, in fact, my favourite people, and their wives, so often acting as animals' nurses, bookkeepers, and general factotums, are the salt of the earth.

Not many veterinarians have taken up the pen to record their varied and interesting lives. Usually they are too busy, or they say they are just incapable of putting it down on paper. Some of them have been kind enough to say that they envied my ability to do this. Well, I don't know about that, but I do know that I envied the gifted RMM when I first opened a book of his cartoons. In fact, I read it in a kind of ecstasy. I just could not believe that these hundreds of brilliant drawings, going right to the heart of our work, could possibly be produced by a man who had to cope with the twenty-four-hours-a-day, seven-days-a-week life I knew so well. With what I can only call a uniquely perceptive genius, he touches on every slant and facet of our profession, and I literally rolled about in my chair, punctuating the belly laughs with gasps of 'Oh yes, that happened to me!' And sometimes, wiping my eyes, I had to admit that even after my forty years at the game, his intuitive skills could still conjure up some aspect that had escaped me. The whole vast spectrum of the veterinary scene is revealed. Apparently effortlessly evoked by a few quick flicks of the pen. The grumpy farmer, the lethal patient, the pampered pets with their whacky, unreasonable owners – they are all there, real, vivid, leaping alive from the pages.

My response to that first book was not only emotional, it was visceral. These things touched me so deeply. They not only made me laugh, they filled me with a warm reassurance that there was somebody far away who had been through it all and had not let the things go by, but had lifted them from his life and preserved them for others to see. It's a funny thing, but much as I love my professional colleagues, the things I like to hear at our get-togethers are not about their impressive and daunting triumphs, but about their embarrassing moments, their awkward predicaments. These are the things that prove we are all fallible, and they comfort me.

When I first took up the manuscript of *Most of My Patients Are Animals*, I wondered – could this man possibly weave his spells in another medium? Within a few pages I realized he was twice blessed, and I began to revel in his stories with the same joy I had felt with the cartoon books. Bob Miller writes beautifully, and I was borne along on waves of clean, uncluttered prose, laughing helplessly most of the time. There were other bonuses, too. In this book I learned something of his personal life, and I found that he dealt with the serious and sometimes tragic incidents with the same sure touch he revealed in the humorous ones. My long held conviction that Dr Miller is a genius is confirmed by this book for all time.

The mixture is incomparably rich. Birds and bulls, horses, sheep and cats. Dogs, cows, monkeys, mules, foxes, bears and lions. I cannot name them all, but Bob Miller has treated them, and as I read, I reacted with the same incredulous delight as before. The man can do just the same with the words as he does with the pictures, and through it all runs the strong thread of his love for his marvellous profession. He can write chillingly, too. He has made me afraid of chimps, and I have never had anything to do with those creatures!

Most of My Patients Are Animals is a lovely panorama of the veterinary scene, but it is not only for our profession, it is for the whole animal-loving world. This picture of a fine man doing his job with dedication, compassion, and good humour will find a response in the heart of every caring person.

Chapter 1

Springtime brings new life. Grasses green the meadows. New leaves adorn the trees. In California, where I have practised veterinary medicine since 1957, wondrous fields of golden poppies and purple lupins paint the hills. New life blesses the countryside.

My home is in an oak-studded canyon. I see a doe with twin fawns. A litter of coyote pups visits my pasture and yodels as darkness falls. The city dwellers know that springtime brings baby animals. They drive into the country to let their children see the young creatures – infant calves, lambs, and kids. Foals pursue their dams on legs too long but with a grace promising future speed and agility.

To a veterinarian – if he is a country practitioner – springtime means dystocia. The British spell it dystokia. The word simply means difficult labour. And labour it is! Labour for the cow or mare trying to bring forth an improperly positioned offspring. Labour for the veterinarian stripped to the waist, with his scrubbed and lubricated arms inserted to the shoulder into the uterus of the straining dam, trying to straighten out the contorted extremities of the unborn young.

We wince when the calls come. Most of them come during the night if the practice includes a lot of horses, as ours does. Mares usually foal at night. When a mare is in trouble foaling, she is in big trouble indeed. Prolonged dystocia usually means the death of the foal, and the contractile powers of the mare are so great that an unrelieved dystocia often causes serious or fatal injury to the mare.

Large-animal obstetrics is, therefore, a routine but difficult part of practice. It is routine because it is common, especially during those spring months when most births occur.

I started our practice, the Conejo Valley Veterinary Clinic. I was the first veterinarian to conduct a private practice in the valley, although one of the larger ranches did have its own full-time resident vet. In those days, the Conejo Valley was a lovely pastoral place, a sea of grass with the groves of ancient oak trees in the washes and along the creeks, surrounded by the rugged, picturesque mountains where I have now taken refuge. There were two little towns in the valley: century-old Newbury Park, a former stagecoach stop, and Thousand Oaks, which came into existence during the twentieth century as a highway town and centre for breeding and training wild animals. The total population was 3,500.

Today, nearly 100,000 people inhabit the area – a part of California's incomparable and almost incomprehensible growth. We have a new city in the valley – Westlake Village, a beautiful, planned community built from scratch. It occupies what was, only a few years ago, a magnificent cattle ranch. Since Spanish colonization, cattle had watered at Triunfo Creek. Now the creek has been dammed to form a man-made lake lined with weeping willows and gracious homes, and dotted with sailboats.

As the area grew, my practice grew. And grew. There are ten veterinarians now in the practice.

At first I worked out of my car. I equipped my station wagon for large-animal calls, and I had a black physician's bag for dogs and cats. I saw them at home and even did major surgery at their homes.

For fifteen years I spent half my time at small-animal practice in the hospital we eventually established, and the other half in the field treating livestock and horses. We also treated many zoo animals.

Gradually, the demands of a growing horse practice led

me to devote nearly all of my time to that speciality. I miss small-animal practice. Occasionally I help out in the hospital, and I enjoy it greatly. I still see zoo species in the field, although more of them are seen at the hospital by my associates.

Subdivisions and suburbanization have greatly reduced our cattle population, so I do not see as many cattle these days. Of course, there are occasional sheep or pigs or goats or camels or tigers or guanacos, but our large-animal practice is mostly equine.

Horses have always been my great and consuming love, so I am quite happy, especially since most of the horses I see are fine, well-bred individuals, primarily thoroughbreds, Arabians, and western breeds.

From a veterinary viewpoint, Thousand Oaks is uniquely situated. Drive fifteen miles in one direction and you are in the suburbs of Los Angeles. Our practice here is a world of show-horse stables, affluent homes surrounded by white fences enclosing valuable horses, and not-so-affluent little homes with fences sometimes made of old bed springs enclosing not-so-valuable horses. Drive in the opposite direction and you are in the farming country of Ventura County, a land of citrus and avocado groves, irrigated pastures, and rolling rangelands. Here we treat pastured horses, cattle, and other farm animals.

Our clients include actors and cowboys, lawyers and tractor drivers, hippies and retired navy personnel, poets, circus performers, and prison guards. We live in a social, ethnic, and cultural melting pot, and it is fascinating.

On a bright May afternoon in 1977 I was called to assist a valuable Arabian mare suffering dystocia. The ranch was in an area being subdivided, and the mare was in a pasture close to the road. The owner was not at home, and I had been called by an inexperienced and thoroughly frightened friend. After disinfecting obstetrical instruments, I scrubbed up and examined the mare.

She was in pain and difficult to restrain. The foal's head

was tucked between its front legs and twisted completely around. One of its front feet and one of its hind feet were protruding from the mare's vagina. While the mare strained mightily, I futilely attempted to push the foal back into the uterus so that I could rearrange its extremities.

Across the road from the ranch was a subdivision. Children were coming home from school. Soon parents and children lined the fence along the road. Parents ran home to bring children to witness a miracle of nature. Children ran home to bring parents to see the spectacle. Cars stopped along the road. Traffic piled up. Police cars arrived. People soon lined three sides of the pasture. Cameras clicked. People took motion pictures. Motorcyclists roared up. 'Hey Mike, get a load of this!'

With the help of a tranquillizer and an epidural anaesthetic, I was able to repel the hind leg. But although I had been working desperately for more than half an hour, I could not recover the missing forelimb, nor could I straighten the contorted neck.

It is rarely necessary to perform a fetotomy on a mare, and I shuddered as I considered sacrificing the still live foal to save the mare. 'Let's see, if I sever the head and get it out of my way, perhaps I can bring that left leg up and get this foal out of there.' I considered doing a caesarean section and rejected the idea. The mare was exhausted. So was I, for that matter. I strained and grunted and sweated and tried. 'My God,' I thought, 'will I have to cut this foal up and deliver it piecemeal in front of all these people? All these children?'

More than a hundred people watched my efforts. I was too anguished to look at their faces. If only we could get the mare up to the barn, away from their sight. But the mare could barely stand. In fact, she went down twice. And the barn was hundreds of yards away, up a hill too steep to drive and across a narrow bridge.

Finally I withdrew my numb and aching arm. I stood dejectedly looking at the ground, resting and thinking. Flash bulbs popped. It was dusk. More cars stopped.

Newer members of the audience made sympathetic sounds as older members brought them up to date. 'Aaah!'

I glanced at my assistant. 'What are you going to do?' he asked.

'I don't know,' I said sadly. 'Try again!'

I tried again. This time I found the missing foreleg. With difficulty I snugged an obstetrical chain around the pastern. Later I found the foal's nose. With my thumb and forefinger in its nostrils, I held it with a death grip. I manipulated the head and neck around into a normal presentation position. The foal was huge – too big for the mare.

With great effort we started to extract the foal. 'We need a man to help pull,' said my assistant. Several men quickly scaled the fence and volunteered. A few minutes later a living, breathing foal lay behind the exhausted but saved mare. We attended both mare and foal. When I finally stood up and gratefully looked at the crowd behind the fence, they broke into applause. Filled with relief, I did a comical little bow.

The foal attempted to stand. Dozens of women and children said, 'Aaaaah!'

A man came forward. He extended his hand. 'You did a wonderful thing,' he said. 'I never saw anything born before, and she was in such terrible trouble. I'll never forget this as long as I live. My daughter here saw it. It was an amazing thing, what you did!'

'It wasn't that special,' I said. 'Really! Just a routine OB. A dystocia. It was routine.'

And I was right. It was routine. It was just a routine dystocia!

But the man was right too. It *was* wonderful. I had done a marvellous thing. I saved the mare and the foal, and I had not realized how wonderful it was. There was the pity of it. Because the work had become routine, I was no longer aware that it was wonderful.

I felt ashamed. To participate in the exciting, marvellous things that veterinarians do every day of their lives and not to realize that they were exciting and marvellous – that was a tragedy.

For twenty years I had been treating 'routine' cases like this dystocia. It took a crowd of city people to make me realize that there are no routine cases and to vow that there would never again be a routine case for me. That is when I decided that, first chance I got, I would sit down and write about it.

Chapter 2

At eighteen years of age I was an infantryman, and the Second World War was nearing its end. When I returned from overseas duty, I entered the University of Arizona under the GI Bill. My major was animal husbandry, in the College of Agriculture.

All during my youth I had devoured books about animals. Stories about horses and dogs, by writers like Will James and Albert Payson Terhune, were my favourite reading.

The hero of my adolescent years was Carl Akeley. Naturalist, artist, author, explorer, and taxidermist, Carl Akeley and his wife, Mary, made many expeditions to Africa, collecting specimens for America's greatest museums. Akeley developed the art of modern taxidermy, mounting animals in lifelike poses and surrounding them with realistic vegetation accurately portrayed, and with birds and smaller animals indigenous to the region. I read and re-read the Akeley books many times. *Brightest Africa,*

The Lion Is A Gentleman and *Lions, Gorillas and Their Neighbors* vividly impressed my boyhood imagination. I wanted nothing more than to spend my life as Akeley had, studying animals, living close to them, and seeing their behaviour in the wild.

Mecca to me was Akeley Hall in the American Museum of Natural History, in New York City. There, to this day, one may see Akeley's marvellous craftsmanship in a hall full of beautifully mounted animal groups. There, too, one may view Akeley's superb life-sized bronzes. At the entrance to the hall is the sculpted work that moved me greatly the first time I viewed it. In it a group of Masai warriors face charging lions.

By the time I was sixteen, however, I realized that the Africa that Akeley knew was fast disappearing. He had been the right man, at the right time in history, and my life was going to be different. Just so long as I worked with animals. After school I worked in a pet shop and a kennel. I spent my summers working on farms, milking cows, and harnessing and driving draught horses. I had read Akeley's books so many times that I had acquired a working knowledge of Swahili from the glossaries in the back, but I had decided to study agriculture. I was a city boy, but I wanted to work with animals.

During the post-war summers I found jobs on ranches, first as a horse wrangler, then as a cowboy, and finally as a horsebreaker. The more I worked with horses, the more I loved them. And the more I became convinced that I wanted to be around animals.

It is said that the most difficult professional school for a student to gain admission to today is the school of veterinary medicine. Well, it was not easy immediately after World War II either. The scholastic excellence now required was not demanded then, but the competition was keen due to the large number of veterans applying for admission.

Getting through veterinary school was relatively easy for

17

me. Getting into the school was another matter. Although I applied to almost every school in the country, my sights were set on Colorado A&M, now Colorado State University. I was an Arizona resident, and Colorado was the closest school. I loved the Rocky Mountain West.

My first application to veterinary school, after one year of undergraduate work, was turned down because a second year of preprofessional curriculum had just been added to the requirements. I applied again the next year, but was told that I needed additional maths courses. The year after that I was again denied admission. My grade average, it was pointed out, was not as high as it should be. In my final preveterinary year, I turned down a position on my school's intercollegiate livestock judging team in order to concentrate on my studies. I made straight A's that year, raising my grade average to a high B. But it got me nowhere.

Bachelor's degree in hand, I decided to move to Colorado and establish residency there, not only to enhance my chances for admission, but also because I planned, at that time, to reside forever in that skier's paradise.

On my day off from work, I visited the campus at Fort Collins and talked to the Dean of the School of Veterinary Medicine.

'Is there anything I can do to enhance my chances of getting into the veterinary school?' I asked. 'I am establishing residency in this state and am working for the Denver County Veterinarian.'

The dean was actually a benevolent, personable man, but he looked alarmingly like J. Edgar Hoover, which did little to quell my apprehension.

He looked at my records, and then asked, 'Why didn't you come up for your interview?'

'I wasn't invited,' I answered, surprised at his question.

'You didn't get a letter asking you to come up for an interview?'

'No, Sir.'

'Alice!' the dean boomed.

18

A venerable secretary appeared.

'Why wasn't Mister Miller asked to come up for an interview? He was selected as an applicant!'

Alice perused my records, and then explained that a mistake had been made – an omission.

Now, I was thrilled, in fact ecstatic, to learn that I had even been considered. While I gloated over this good news, I suddenly realized the dean was speaking.

'. . .terribly sorry about this unfortunate incident. We have already selected the class for the coming school year, but perhaps we can interview you here and now, and you may qualify as an alternate for that class.'

'An interview?' I responded. 'Now?'

'Yes,' he said. 'I'll call the committee together immediately.'

He bustled out to gather the inquisitors while I fought rising panic. I was not ready for an interview that day. I had not prepared myself psychologically. Adrenalin flowed. My hands shook. I noted that my shoes were not shined. I fled to the restroom, removed my undershorts, and buffed my shoes with them with manic vigour, convinced that my future depended upon their appearance, a concept probably incomprehensible to today's youth.

My mouth was so dry I could barely speak or swallow. I drank from the rest room faucet.

Trembling with fear, I returned to the dean's office to face the admissions committee.

The three men who sat there looked, at the time, like the three coldest, most impassive human beings I had ever seen.

There was the dean, J. Edgar Hoover. Dean Floyd Cross, whom I later learned was as kind and sweet a gentleman as ever lived, held his cigarette habitually between his thumb and forefinger, with his palm up. The cigarette pointed outwards, and he puffed at the end nearest his palm. The only person I had seen smoke like that was an SS officer in a World War II movie. He was the one who said, just before he tortured the girl, 'Ve haf vays

19

to make you talk!'

The second member of the committee was head of the bacteriology department, Doctor Deem. I learned later what a gentle, decent man he was. But at that moment, all I could see was his lean aquiline features, his furrowed cheeks (duelling scars?) and – no eyes! That's right! He sat facing the window, and the light reflected in his rimless glasses concealed his eyes. It had the same effect the mirrored sunglasses of the motorcycle policeman have.

My terror turned to hysteria as I turned pitifully toward the third and last member of the committee. Perhaps here I would find a kindly academic countenance. No! Doctor Rue Jensen stood there, looking at me grimly. Later, Doctor Jensen was to be one of the teachers I respected most. But now I saw a short, muscular man, the blue shadow of a heavy beard on his cruel face. His hair was cropped short in a crew cut. His arms were sinewy, and in one hand he held – a great, gleaming, razor-sharp cleaver!

Dr Jensen, a pathologist who had been on his way to the autopsy room to cleave a cow, put his cleaver aside. The interview began.

I was so nervous I could hardly speak. I had difficulty concentrating on their questions. Once, I thought I heard screams in the basement.

Then Dr Deem did something so simple, so earthy, so American, so rural that I almost smiled, and I began to relax. He pulled out a brown cigarette paper and a can of Prince Albert, and rolled himself a smoke.

I was not accepted that year. No alternate was needed. But I did get in the following year. I was on my way toward becoming a veterinarian. Of all the difficulties that route entailed, none was as momentarily intimidating as that day back in 1951 when I faced the admissions committee in Colorado.

'Congratulations,' said the penny postcard, 'upon your acceptance to the Colorado A&M School of Veterinary Medicine. I am a veterinary student and own a house with

20

rooming facilities. Most of our tenants are veterinary or preveterinary students. If you would like to reserve a place, please contact me. The rates are $12.50 per month.'

I reserved a spot on what was later to be called The Stud Farm, and I lived there through four years of veterinary education. I can still remember how we protested when, during my final year, the rent was raised to $13.50 per month. A dollar in 1952 bought a luxurious dinner in Fort Collins, Colorado.

Tenants at The Stud Farm lived in the basement, the horse barn, and one even resided in the chicken coop. The horse barn had rooms in what had been the hayloft, and other rooms in the stable area. There was one shower and a sink for the entire barn, which housed nine or ten men. The man in the chicken coop also used our sink and shower.

The room in which I lived was a large one. It had, I suspect, been a foaling stall. It accommodated three students, each on an army-surplus bunk with springs made of clothesline. There was a rug on the floor. When the wind blew, the rug would balloon up off the floor. Under the rug one could find oats and ancient bits of hay. The ceiling planks formed the floor of the hayloft. These planks had shrunk with age, and one could see, through the cracks between the boards, the feet of the boys who lived upstairs. If anyone up there spilled coffee, it dripped on us. In reprisal we would load a hypodermic syringe with ink and squirt it through the cracks in the ceiling. The objective was to stain the socks of the unsuspecting man above.

There was a gas heater in the room, but not being suicidal, we turned it off at night and crawled beneath mounds of old army blankets. When it was twenty degrees below zero outside, the temperature in our room would drop to ten above. Fortunately, such temperatures are infrequent in Fort Collins.

College days, the annual spring campus celebration, was highlighted by a parade and an intercollegiate rodeo. There was also a Whiskerino Contest. The contest winner, in those smooth-shaven and crew-cut college days, was he who grew the most luxurious and striking beard.

Jack was a freshman preveterinary student. He lived at The Stud Farm when I was in my third year of veterinary medicine. As College Days approached, Jack stopped indulging in his once-a-week shave. After several weeks, a fungoid fuzz adorned his chin and upper lip. One night we veterinary students came home late from a meeting. Jack greeted us and said, 'Hey, you guys know all about drugs. Is there something that will stimulate the growth of hair?'

'Certainly,' I said. 'We use a special formula to encourage the growth of hair on show cattle. Why?' My fellow students, immediately sensing an opportunity, nodded in agreement.

'It's call Hair-Suit,' one offered inventively.

Jack dug his toe into the rug, stirring some oats around, and confessed, 'It's this beard! I grew it for the Whiskerino Contest, but as you can see, I'm not going to have much to show for the effort. I thought if you guys knew of something. . .'

'Say no more,' said Val Farrel. 'We'll go right back to the pharmacy and get some for you!'

'Gee,' said Jack, 'I hate to impose on you, but I sure would appreciate it!'

At midnight Val and I went back to the hospital. We filled an ointment tin with a depilatory cream used to remove the hair from rabbits before they underwent abdominal surgery. We added a bit of methylene blue dye. We labelled it Hair Suit and added, 'To stimulate hair growth, massage in cream, leave ten minutes, and then wash off with soap and water.'

Jack was asleep when we got back, but the next afternoon, alerted to what was to transpire, the whole Stud Farm had gathered in my room under the pretext of having a country music festival. While guitars strummed and a fiddle squealed, Jack appeared.

Given the 'hair grower,' Jack smeared the blue ointment all over his face and worked it in while we pretended to ignore him, choking back laughter. When he went to the lone hallway sink to remove the cream, we crowded after him. He diligently lathered a wash rag and wiped away the cream. His beard and moustache came with it. All that was left was his smooth skin, dyed blue.

Several days passed. Then Jack came to see me. 'I can see the humour in the prank you fellows pulled on me,' he said. 'No hard feelings. My beard was a failure anyway.' Then a tear glistened in his eye. 'But I don't want to go through life without a beard. Isn't there any kind of an antidote for that stuff?'

That night I conferred with my cohorts. 'Jack thinks his beard is lost permanently,' I explained. 'He wants an antidote.'

'He has a right to an antidote!' exclaimed Gene Taylor. 'Let's give him a solution of silver nitrate. If he applies it indoors, then goes out in the sun, his skin will turn black.'

Saturday afternoon our gang, including Jack, went to the Dew Drop Inn, a local joint that served 3.2 beer. There, in the dim recesses of a corner booth, we quaffed and joked and fraternized while jack dutifully applied the silver nitrate to his face. The label read 'To restore hair growth, apply like shaving lotion every hour.'

As we walked home later, we were disappointed to note that Jack's face looked the same: basic pink with a faint methylene blue tint. Apparently our silver nitrate solution was too weak. However, we were soon heartened by Jack's surprised voice. 'Hey, my fingernails are all brown!'

'Oh, Oh!' I stepped back, wiping my hands on my pants. 'It's paronychia pigmentosa!'

My associates recoiled in horror.

'Paronychia pigmentosa? My God! That's the earliest sign of Rocky Mountain leprosy!'

Jack looked at us sideways, and then sneered, 'Come on, you guys! You must think I'm gullible!'

Chapter 3

I was no longer a youth. I had been a bachelor and a student for a long time, but in my senior year of veterinary school, both of those roles were about to end. I would soon be a graduate veterinarian, a doctor of veterinary medicine, and I would soon be a married man. During my final year, I met Debby, who was one of 700 women students at Colorado A&M. I had noticed her on campus that year – a pretty, shy girl with a sweet smile, short dark hair, and long shapely legs, but she looked so young that I assumed she was a freshman. After all, could a senior veterinary student, a war veteran, date a freshman girl?

At a college rodeo, I watched her ride in the women's barrel race. A formidable competitor, she rode aggressively, one with the big quarter horse gelding, a roping horse she had borrowed and taught to run the barrels. I learned too that she was a senior student, twenty-three years of age, and had transferred from a Texas school to compete on Colorado's national champion collegiate rodeo team. When I asked her for a date, she accepted, and a romance bloomed. We learned that we had important compatibilities. We both had an overwhelming love for animals. We both loved the out-of-doors, riding, skiing, and being close to nature. We shared a philosophy of a life of gentleness, of kindness to our fellow man and other living things, of tolerance for other people's values, and a fascination for other cultures.

Debby's father was a physician – a general practitioner whose entire life had been devoted to his practice. She knew, better than I, the demands of medical practice, its rigours, its unrelenting hours, and the perversities of the public the practitioner served. She viewed marriage to a country veterinarian with some apprehension, but nevertheless, we were married soon after graduation. Our love of animals has been an important bond over the years.

Our life has been filled with an abundance of dogs, cats, mules, horses, ponies, and goats.

It is good that veterinarians' wives love animals. How could they otherwise tolerate the irregular hours, the late dinners, and the nights, weekends, and holidays with a husband on call unless they empathized with the sick and injured creatures needing their husband's skill? But sometimes this love of animals can be carried too far. Debby, for example, has a special affinity for injured animals lying along the highway.

Shortly after we were married, she gasped as we were driving one day and said, 'Did you see that?'

'What?'

'That black dog lying by the shoulder. It was run over!'

'Was it alive?'

'I don't know. I think so. It looked like it was breathing. Let's go back.'

I turned the car around.

'It looked like a Labrador retriever.'

We drove back only to find a discarded black inner tube.

'I don't think I can save it,' I said.

Over the years, I have turned back to aid a score or more inner tubes. Most were damaged beyond help.

Wild animals hit by automobiles are also the object of Debby's compassion. A typical scene goes like this:

'Oh, no!' Debby exclaims.

'What did you see?' I ask.

'A coyote, poor thing, hit on the highway!'

'Yes, I saw it.'

'Do you think it was still alive?'

'No, it was dead.'

'How can you be sure?'

'It was flat and red.'

'But how do you know it was dead?'

'If it were alive it would have snapped at the buzzards. Didn't you see six or seven buzzards all around the top of the coyote?'

'Yes!' Then, after a long pause, 'I think one of the

buzzards had a broken wing.'

On one occasion, we simultaneously spotted a yellow cat by the side of the road. It was supporting its weight on its front legs, hind legs awkwardly drawn forward, and it had a hump in its back.

'Did you see that poor cat?' cried Debby.

'Yes. It must have just been hit. Looks like its back or pelvis has been broken.'

I turned the car around and reached the cat just as it finished its bowel movement. It covered the faeces with sand, stared at us hostilely, and disappeared into a culvert.

The most humiliating of these roadside Samaritan adventures occurred when my wife screamed, 'Oh, Bob, stop the car! It's a collie, and he's still alive!'

'Are you sure? Maybe it was a sable-and-white inner tube.'

'No, please! I saw it! A collie! And it moved. It's alive!'

Wearily I stopped and backed up several hundred yards to find a hippy, with a long mane and shaggy blond beard. He was curled up roadside, stoned into oblivion, fifty miles from the closest town.

'I told you it wasn't an inner tube,' said Debby. 'I was partly right.'

'You were also partly wrong.' I pointed out. 'You said it was alive. I think it's been dead a long time!'

'Yes,' she agreed. 'It smells badly decomposed.'

Chapter 4

After we had graduated and been married, Debby and I moved down to Arizona, my previous home. There we discovered an old adobe house on a ranch east of Tucson. I was employed at an animal hospital not too many miles away, and we were happy to find the snug little house for rent. It had been the original ranch house on this working ranch, and the new owner had built a sumptuous new residence for himself.

There were several other homes on the place. In one of them, next to the adobe we had rented, an old vaquero, Enrico, lived in retirement. His life had been spent working for this ranch, and the new owner had kindly let him continue to live there. He spent his days dozing in the sun, or in the shade, depending upon the temperature.

Our house had no heating system, only a fireplace in the living room and the oven in the kitchen stove. The oven, like Enrico, the ranch, and the adobe, was venerable. I carried my bride, Debby, over the threshold in September. The mornings were still warm, so we had no occasion to light the oven. After a few days, Debby decided to bake. I was away working when she lit the match. The explosion blew the oven door apart. Debby wasn't hurt, but her face was blackened. She ran outside. Enrico sat next door, rocking.

'The oven!' Debby cried. 'It exploded! Did you hear it? It blew up!' She gesticulated excitedly.

Enrico beamed at her. His few remaining teeth, either snaggled or gleaming gold, were revealed by his broad smile.

'Si!' He nodded. 'Eet's a nice day!'

Our next home was even less prepossessing. When we moved to Thousand Oaks, California, that sleepy little village had two places available to us. There were log cabins

27

at the Redwood Lodge Motel and a garage in town that had been converted to a one-room apartment. The motel wouldn't allow pets, so Debby and I and our Australian shepherd dog, Wendy, a crippled and nearly hairless former patient we had acquired in Arizona, moved into the garage.

We stored our things in boxes under the bed. As a result, the legs of the bed were off the floor. In one corner, a curtained-off area served as a bathroom. In another corner, a sink and an old stove marked the kitchen area. The stove looked remarkably like the one that blew up in Arizona.

'When are you going to use the oven?' I asked Debby after a few weeks.

'I'm afraid to light it,' she admitted.

'I'll light it,' I offered.

I used up a box of kitchen matches before I learned the trick. The secret was to turn on the gas, wait ten seconds (I would count, 'one thousand one, one thousand two, one thousand three,' and so on) and then drop a lighted match into a hole over the burner. The oven would then ignite, with a soft 'whomp.'

After a year in the garage, we bought a little house. It leaked badly in the rain, but it had a yard for our dog, a pasture for our horse, and an oven with a pilot light that worked perfectly.

Mr Moore, our former landlord, came out to see me one day while I was on a call next door to see a neighbour's horse.

'Good to see you, Doctor,' he said. 'I hope you and Mrs Miller are happy in your new home. I'd like to ask a favour of you. I rented the garage to an elderly couple after you moved out. They don't know how to light the oven, and I haven't been able to figure it out either. I remember that you had a system. When you've finished with the horse, would you mind coming over to show us how?'

'Sure,' I agreed, and as soon as my call was completed I went next door. Mr Moore introduced me to a white-haired couple in their eighties.

'Daddy can't survive without his biscuits,' the old lady explained, 'but I can't light the danged oven!'

Her husband added wrathfully, 'Ain't had biscuits since I moved! I've got to have biscuits with my morning coffee!'

'It's simple!' I said. 'It took me a while to find the right combination, but once I learned, it never failed.'

The old man took out a match.

'Turn on the gas,' I suggested.

He turned on the gas.

'Now don't light it immediately. The gas will blow the match out,' I explained. 'Wait ten seconds and then light it.'

'Ten seconds?' he asked.

'Yes,' I answered, 'count to ten!'

'One, two, three, four. . .'

'No, no!' I corrected him. 'Not so fast! Count seconds, like this, a thousand one, a thousand two, a thousand. . .'

'What?' the old man demanded. 'A thousand seconds? What are you talking about?'

'No,' I explained patiently while the gas hissed. 'You say a thousand one, a thousand two to count the seconds.'

'Why can't I use my watch?' he demanded.

'Okay, fine!' I agreed. 'Use your watch!'

The old man fumbled for his watch, adjusted his bifocals, and started to count, 'One, two, three. . .'

When he came to ten, I said, 'Now! Now light the oven!'

'Now?' he asked.

'Yes!' I said. As we both peered into the oven, he struck a match.

The blast threw us both back against the wall. Mr Moore and the old lady, on either side of us, recoiled in terror. For a moment there was a stunned silence. The oven was lit. The hair on my arms was singed. I looked at the old man. His glasses were askew.

'Well,' he gasped, 'to hell with the damned biscuits!'

Chapter 5

Debby and I had roamed California, looking for a place to set up practice. As we entered the Conejo Valley on Highway 101, I was captivated by the beauty I saw. Here was a valley of grasslands, green and undulating in the March wind. Gnarled and sturdy oak trees lined the draws and studded the rolling foothills, and the horizon was lined with dark mountain peaks. Beautiful horses – thoroughbreds, standardbreds, and quarter horses – ran in white fenced pastures, and everywhere, in all directions, fat cattle grazed in the fields.

Conejo means *rabbit* in Spanish, and the valley was nicknamed for its abundant rabbits, but the original name for the area, assigned by the early Spanish as they ascended to that plateau from sea-level, was *Las Altagracias* – the graceful highlands. How well named this valley was, this gentle and pastoral place. How far removed it seemed from burgeoning Los Angeles, only an hour's drive away.

The Camino Real – the King's Highway – the original Mission trail developed by the early Spanish ran the length of the valley, connecting the San Fernando Valley of Los Angeles with San Francisco, four hundred miles to the North.

Thousand Oaks had motels and restaurants lining the old highway, forming a single, twisting main street several miles long. It was an unincorporated, shabby, misshapen community that had grown up to dominate the Conejo Valley, with a population of twelve hundred souls, but it was not the town itself that attracted Debby and me to the area. It was the valley, rich in livestock and horses, but even more exciting, as we drove through the village, was a great barn labelled 'Louis Goebel – Importer and Exporter of Wild Animals.' I saw a garishly painted 'World Jungle Compound' and a sign that read 'Lion Farm'. There were circus wagons parked in empty lots. Elephants were staked in fields, lions and tigers chained to oak trees.

'Jungleland!' declared a sign. 'Admission One Dollar. See Wild Animal Movie Stars.'

I was thirty years of age, recently married, broke, and out of a job, but I had come home.

We found a telephone book, a slender volume of just a few pages marked 'Thousand Oaks, Newbury Park, Lake Sherwood and Surrounding Communities.' There were only 3,500 people in the entire valley. I turned to the yellow pages at the back of the book and looked under 'Veterinarians.' The only names listed were in communities outside the area. The Conejo Valley had no practising veterinarian.

'This is the place!' I said to Debby.

'Yes,' she said. 'This looks like the right place.'

One Saturday night, after we had lived in Thousand Oaks for a few months, a community dance was held in a circus tent, set up on the Jungleland parking lot. I marvelled at the unusual variety of townspeople. There were the Jungleland and circus folk, the ordinary variety of small-town people, a sprinkling of writers and a movie director from Lake Sherwood, a couple of film stars who owned ranches in the valley, cowboys from the horse farms and cattle ranches, and hillbilly types, some of whom lived in run-down town residences, and others who had come down from the hills. The crowd included movie star Joel McCrea, cowboys Gerald Davis and Buster Naegele, horsewoman Belle Holloway, horseshoer Pete Kelley, cattleman Bob Elders, tiger trainer Mabel Stark, and, of course, many others. As Debby and I looked at the colourful residents of Thousand Oaks, she said, 'I wonder if there is another town with such an assortment of characters?'

Suddenly I realized that this was our town, the community we had chosen to live in, to build a practice in, to grow with, to rear children in; where we could work with animals and their owners for the rest of our lives. We were young and hopeful, and oh what adventures lay ahead.

Having read Carl Akeley's *Lion Country* many times, I

31

was familiar with the night time roaring pattern of the African lion. Now, living in Thousand Oaks, I thrilled nightly to one of nature's most stirring serenades. Forty African lions resided at Jungleland, a few short blocks from our home. The roaring, as Akeley described, began softly, each roar louder and stronger than the preceding, a rhythmic ritual that evoked some primeval memory in my being, because as the sound of forty lions roaring in chorus reached a crescendo, the adrenalin coursed through my body, and I was wide awake from a deep sleep. The crescendo having been reached, the roars rapidly diminished in volume and in length, finally terminated in a soft coughing sound. The boyhood dreams Akeley's books had inspired in me years before, of listening to the sounds of the veldt from a safari tent, were being realized in my new California veterinary practice. Daily I worked not only with domestic animals, but with exotic species of all kinds.

Once when I came home of an evening I found a truckload of ostriches parked in front of my house.

Another time a large male orangutang escaped from Jungleland one night and made its way to the back door of a neighbour's home. It tapped softly at the door. The lady of the house, answering the knock, was appalled to find herself facing a 400-pound pot-bellied demon covered with long red hair. Slamming the door and locking it, she hysterically telephoned for my assistance, but before I arrived the demonic looking but gentle orang had been docilely led home by Jungleland personnel.

Not long after we had settled down, we acquired a second dog, an egomaniacal dalmation named Keno. Keno was the self-appointed guardian of our property, and a ring of the doorbell brought him to the door with ferocious enthusiasm. Toenails clattering on the linoleum, breathlessly barking his outrage, Keno would sprint to the front of the house, and when we opened the door an inch or two to see who was there, he would rave and shriek and try to force his bulk through the crack. Normally we would ask the caller to wait while we put the dog out in the back yard.

One evening, as Debby and I sat watching television, the doorbell rang. Keno leaped up and attempted to hurtle towards the door, barking savagely. Due to the slippery linoleum on the floor, he accelerated gradually, even though he was running at top speed. Consequently, we both reached the door at the same time. Opening it a crack, I started to lean forward to peek out and see who was there. Keno abruptly stopped barking, whined, and putting his head down and his tail between his legs, retreated to the corner with an expression of apprehensive embarrassment on his face. Puzzled, I opened the door. There stood Ralph Helfer, later to become a well-known wild animal trainer in the entertainment world. The young man held a leash at the end of which was a full grown African lion. 'I got a sick lion,' he said, 'is the doctor in?'

The lion recovered, and he too became famous – the star of a motion picture, 'Clarence the Cross-Eyed Lion.'

Chapter 6

I am a sound sleeper, so I did not immediately wake up when the telephone rang, even though it was close to my head. Debby jabbed me and sleepily mumbled 'telephone' in my ear as it rang for the second time.

'This is Colonel Thornton,' a distraught voice said. 'Prince is worse. I can't get him up any more.'

Twenty minutes later I drove up to the stable at the Thornton ranch. The light was on in Prince's stall.

'If there is one chance in a million to save this horse, I

want you to try,' said the Colonel. 'He was in the Olympics, you know, before you were born.'

'No, I was already alive during that Olympics, but I would have been too young to remember,' I responded.

'The Colonel looked up at me. The horse's great head was cradled in the Colonel's lap, the muzzle grey, the lips hanging slackly open, revealing gums coloured purple with approaching death, the eyes clouded with pain and toxicity. Colonel Thornton's face looked curiously childlike, streaked with tears.

'He'll be thirty years old next month,' said the Colonel. 'You can't imagine what a great horse this is – what a noble, great horse. I remember him from the Olympics. A three-day horse, that's a gruelling event, you know. I never dreamed he'd be mine. He was given to me a few years ago, and he is remarkable. Still sound! Still willing! Still jumping! Never refuses! Never does anything wrong!'

Colonel Thornton was US Army, retired, a veteran of two wars. It was awkward to see him sitting there in the straw bedding, holding the dying gelding's head, crying like a little boy. Two days earlier, the Colonel had left the feed-room door unlatched, and the horse – I'll call him Prince – had wandered in and eaten his fill. The old fellow was just used as a lesson horse now, to teach children the rudiments of English riding. The Colonel had opened the first English riding school in the Conejo Valley, prematurely, I guess, because it eventually failed financially. Prince, long retired from competition, was so gentle and reliable that he was allowed to wander about the premises at will. That's what he was doing when he found the feed-room door open. During the night the old horse had consumed much of a sack of barley. By the time the Colonel came down to the stable to feed the horses at dawn, old Prince was already rolling on the ground, in pain from colic.

'How much grain did he eat?' was my first question.

'I don't know,' the Colonel answered, anxiously. 'I can't be sure, but it couldn't have been more than twenty-five pounds.'

'Are you sure?' I said. 'It's important?'

'Yes,' said the Colonel. 'Twenty-five pounds! Maybe less!'

'Is he used to grain?' I wanted know.

'Oh yes,' said the Colonel. 'He works every day, and gets at least two pounds at each feeding.'

'Then,' I said, 'we have a chance, but he looks so bad, as if he had consumed a lot more than twenty-five pounds. He really looks bad. Maybe it's his age.'

For the next two days I returned to the stable repeatedly to administer to Prince. I did everything for him that can be done in a case of this kind, but I knew from the start, although like the Colonel I would not admit it, that the old horse was doomed.

By the evening of the first day, he had foundered. In addition to the abdominal distress the poor beast now suffered excruciating pain in his feet, the principal target of the enigmatic disease known as founder.

'It sounds very bad,' I told the Colonel in the middle of the night when he telephoned.

'Please come again,' he had implored. 'He is in terrible pain.' I went and stayed with the suffering horse and the tired, guilt-ridden man until nearly dawn.

'I don't think there is much hope,' I said. 'Even if he were to survive, his feet are ruined. He is in terrible pain. Is it right to let him go this way?'

'Doctor,' the Colonel said quietly, 'I want this horse to live, and if there is a ghost of a chance, I want you to keep on trying. I've been a military man all my life. I don't surrender, and this horse, if he could talk, would tell you that he won't surrender. He's a fighter, as game as any horse I've ever known, and he's like me. We'd rather die than surrender.'

Reluctantly, I went on, doing all I could for Prince, to control his pain, and futilely trying to reverse the process that was destroying his life. Now, after two days of suffering for the horse, the Colonel, and myself, Prince could no longer stand. He no longer thrashed and cramped and rolled with pain. Groaning periodically, he just lay there, with laboured respiration, lips parted, the long old yellow teeth showing. The old warrior was dying.

The Colonel bent over to speak. 'Come on old boy! You can do it! You're not through yet! Oh, what a gallant old man you are! You'll see this through!'

I shook my head. The Colonel was refusing to face up to the situation. He had made a mistake, a novice's mistake, in leaving the feed-room door unlatched. Now, guilt-ridden, he could not admit that his carelessness had led to the imminent death of this horse that he loved.

I put my hand on his shoulder. 'Colonel, it's time to face reality,' I said softly. 'It's time to render your last kindness to this horse. Let's end his pain.'

The Colonel looked up at me. He had not slept for two nights. His eyes were reddened with fatigue and sorrow. He searched my face, and then he said, 'I've always wondered if there is a God. Now, I know! There can't be! God could not let a poor innocent animal suffer this way.'

Then, he buried his face in Prince's mane and broke down, weeping convulsively, like a child. Tears streamed down my own face as I saw this man, a retired officer, commander of men in battle, in this state.

'I'll get the anaesthetic,' I said, patting his shoulder, and went out to my station wagon to get the drug. Before I could finish loading the syringe, however, I heard a wail from inside the stall, and I knew it was all over. Prince had died.

A day later, the Colonel telephoned. 'I want to thank you for your efforts,' he said. 'I spent the morning on the tractor, digging a hole to bury Prince in, down in the pasture, under the oaks. I feel bad about one thing, and I want to own up to it now. When I told you that Prince had not eaten more than twenty-five pounds of grain, I knew that wasn't true. You see, he tore open a full hundred-pound sack of grain, and when I found him in the morning, there was only about twenty-five pounds left in it. I wasn't completely honest with you, as you were with me. I don't know why I didn't tell you the truth, but I want you to know it now.'

Chapter 7

All young veterinarians face similar difficulties when establishing new practices, especially if they're starting out in an unfamiliar area. And in a wide-ranging rural practice, the new doctor has the fundamental problem of simply figuring out how to get where he is going.

Typically I would look over my list of calls for the day, trying to decide where to start. Fred Gibbons, over in the Simi Valley, had a bunch of horses for me to worm. I'd make that my first call and then work my way back to Thousand Oaks. After lunch I could reverse the procedure, starting my calls in Calabasas, and again work my way home.

Fred had just moved to a new place, so I jotted down his address on my call list, 1471 Peach Road. Finding Peach Road was easy, and I drove slowly up the street, scanning the mail boxes for the number 1471 and taking in the unfamiliar territory. There was fifteen-hundred-and-something, followed by an orange grove badly in need of cultivation. The next place had to be Fred's.

I pulled into the driveway and got out of the pickup. Two steps up onto the porch and I knocked on the door.

A young woman answered, her head wrapped in a towel. She peered at me through the door.

'I'm Doctor Miller,' I said, smiling. She must be Fred's

wife, I thought. I'd never met her.

'I was washing my hair,' she explained, poking at the towel with both hands. 'May I help you?'

'I'm Doctor Miller,' I repeated. She cocked her head and squinted at me. She looked puzzled.

'I'm the veterinarian!'

'Yes?'

Surely Fred had told her I was coming. In fact, I expected him to be there to assist me. Still no glimmer of understanding shone in her eyes. She just stood there, behind the screen, with her head wrapped in that silly towel, gaping at me. It was, I thought, a sort of comical situation.

So, I took a step forward, spread my arms in a palms-upward gesture, and said, with a kind of fanfare effect, 'I'm here to kill the worms!'

The effect of my words surprised me. Her hands froze on the towel. Her eyes widened, her lips parted and quivered, and her entire face went pale. The smile left my face. The woman was in shock. She was stunned.

'I'm Doctor Miller, I have an appointment here to worm a bunch of horses. Is Fred home?'

The lady's eyes closed. Relief flooded her expression. One hand left the towel, and she clutched at her throat.

'Oh, my goodness,' she sputtered. 'Oh, my! I think you want the place across the road!'

'Thank you,' I said, frowning at her senseless reaction, and retreated to my truck.

An hour later, as I drove out of Fred's driveway, I saw the sign on the fence across the road. It read: 'The Worm Ranch – International Earthworm Distributors.'

Apparently earthworm farming was an important industry, and it happens that at 1472 Peach Road, directly across from Fred's new quarter horse farm, was one of California's most successful earthworm farms. It shipped great quantities of worms to all parts of the country – in fact, all over the world. The worms, I later learned, were not for fish bait, but for soil improvement.

*

Ultimately, for the new veterinarian, more important than finding the client's house is earning his (or her) confidence – and then keeping it.

I was very fond of old Mr Brossard. Pink cheeked and vivacious in his eighties, the old man lived in a tiny cabin at the edge of town. When he needed groceries he would ride into town on an old sorrel mare. His only other companions were several milk goats and a wonderful old Australian shepherd dog. I thought the world of the loyal old dog, and knowing that Mr Brossard was a pensioner, I used to vaccinate his dog every year free of charge.

One day he telephoned to tell me that his dog had become so decrepit that he felt it should be put to sleep. I told him to bring me the dog and I would put him to sleep at no charge.

'Ain't got transportation, Doc,' he said. 'Can you come to the house to do it? I can't carry him on the horse.'

I somewhat reluctantly agreed to make a house call, knowing that the old man could not afford to pay for the service, and that it would have to be gratis.

The cabin was so small, and it was such a beautiful warm day, that I decided to do the job outside, in front of the house. The old man wanted to bury his companion, but did not want to watch it die. I sympathetically suggested that he go inside while I did what had to be done.

I filled a syringe, put a tourniquet on the old dog's leg and began the injection. Suddenly the dog jerked the leg, and I lost the vein. He had received just enough anaesthetic to put him into the excitatory stage of anaesthesia. Immediately he started to yelp hysterically, meanwhile making wild running movements with his legs.

'Quiet,' I implored. I lay on top of the big dog to hold him down, and held his muzzle closed with one hand to stifle his cries.

The screams continued to emit from the corners of his mouth, while he urinated all over me. The old man came out of the house.

'What the hell are you doing to Old Blue?' he demanded.

Across the road a lady came out of a house, 'What's he doing to Old Blue?' she yelled.

A teen-age boy on a bicycle stopped and ordered, 'Get off that dog, mister! Let go of that dog!'

I let go. The running and screaming reached a crescendo. 'Do something!' yelled the old man.

I threw myself back on top of Old Blue. Desperately I tried to hit a vein. Finally I injected the rest of the barbiturate until, after an interminable period of time during which the old man ranted and fumed, 'That's a terrible way to do Old Blue,' the dog lay quiet.

I sadly packed up my things. Other neighbours had gathered now, all silently glaring at me as I wretchedly drove away.

Even if we veterinarians suffer humiliations, they are not all so painful, and if benevolent intentions occasionally backfire, sometimes we are able to set a good example. An enormous Santa Gertrudis cow had a prolapsed uterus. She was so tall that I had to stand on a brick beside the chute in order to inject an epidural anaesthetic into her spine at the base of her tail.

When I arrived, the cow was in the chute. The only person there to assist me was the ranch hand's kid brother. He was nattily attired in a green-and-white soccer uniform. The white portions gleamed. He looked clean and well-scrubbed. I asked him to grasp the cow's tail and lift it while I palpated for the injection site. He gingerly took hold of the tail about two feet from its base.

'Closer,' I said, 'Hold the tail closer to her body.' He reluctantly advanced his hand a few inches. The base of the tail was, of course, coated with manure, and he was obviously trying to avoid touching it.

'Closer,' I said. 'Hold it real close to her body.' His hand advanced another few inches.

'Look,' I said. 'A little manure won't hurt you. Grab her tail right next to her body and lift it.'

With an offended expression on his face, he grasped the

messy tail properly, and I soon completed the injection.

I tied the cow's tail forward, got my equipment ready and stepped into the chute behind the cow. She greeted me by humping her back and ejecting a stream of manure with the explosive force of water from a firehose.

I was caught completely by surprise, and because the cow was so tall, the manure hit me full in the face. I was wearing a cap made of ventilated fabric. Through the mesh, my hair was plastered with manure. My left ear was stuffed full. I couldn't see. Unfortunately, my mouth was open when the explosion occurred. I doubt if my mouth was visible. My coveralls were drenched; gobs of manure ran down inside them.

I wiped my eyes until I could see. My assistant, now positioned at the head of the cow, studied me impassively. He didn't frown. He didn't smile. His face was expressionless. There was a glint in his eyes suggesting that, in school the next morning, this story would be told with great glee. But right now there was nothing.

I wiped my mouth with my right shoulder, which somehow was unspattered.

I matched the youth's expression. I didn't swear. I didn't spit. I didn't react in any way except to clear my vision and my mouth. I looked at him as he looked at me, deadpan.

Then I said, 'See! It looks bad. It smells bad. It tastes bad. But it can't *hurt* you!'

Chapter 8

Pioneering a country veterinary practice in a small town, I wasn't making much money. It was hard to make ends meet.

Debby took a part-time job training cutting horses in the San Fernando Valley. I decided to do some cartooning to supplement my income. I had been drawing cartoons most of my life, and for the most part it only served to get me in trouble with my teachers. I had never tried selling any until I was in veterinary school. During my pre-veterinary college years, I worked part-time washing dishes in the school cafeteria between classes, cutting brush for a surveyor, selling ice cream after school, and working for a veterinarian weekends. Summers I worked as a ranch hand, and during school holidays I worked at whatever I could find, including caddying at a golf course and picking cotton, fruit, and other crops. My GI Bill was saved for veterinary school, a prudent bit of planning because the hours of study required for my medical training didn't allow me to work on the side. Still, I needed extra money, and I started cartooning for ranching and livestock magazines, signing the cartoons 'Bob Miller.'

Now that I was a practising veterinarian, albeit a financially struggling one, I preferred anonymity as a cartoonist and started to sell cartoons to veterinary journals, signing them 'RMM.' The situations I experienced every day served as grist for my cartoon mill. At the time, I intended to cartoon only until my practice income was sufficient to drop the artwork. I could not imagine that the hobby of cartooning would become an avocation leading to the eventual publication of four books of veterinary cartoons. One of the journals I drew for revealed the identity of the anonymous RMM in an article they published without my knowledge, and the secret was out. In nearly thirty years of practice, I have had thousands of cartoons published, and people often ask how I can keep coming up with new ones. 'Why,' I explain, 'I am engaged in the most versatile and unending source of cartoon material that any human activity can provide: the practice of veterinary medicine.' What career offers, every day, such a sublime array of situations as what I do for a living? Life in all its variety parades constantly before the veterinarian. All I need do is observe and absorb the humour, the pathos, and the excitement in what I do.

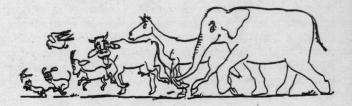

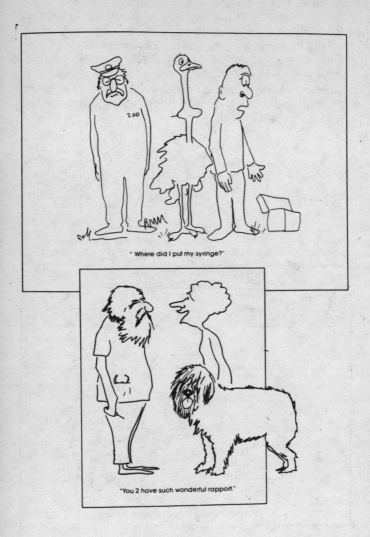

" Where did I put my syringe?"

"You 2 have such wonderful rapport."

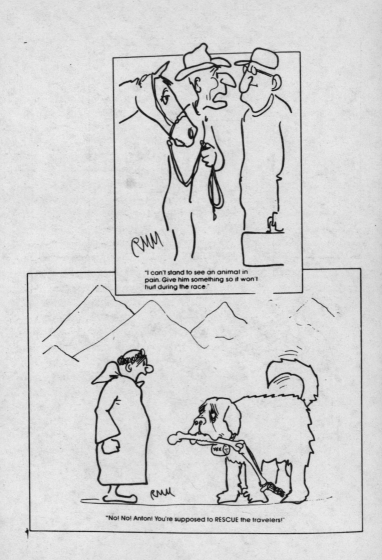

"I can't stand to see an animal in pain. Give him something so it won't hurt during the race."

"No! No! Anton! You're supposed to RESCUE the travelers!"

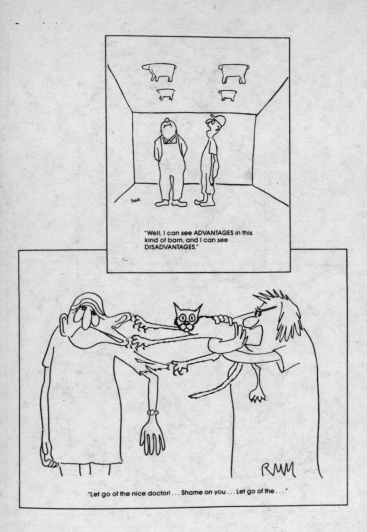

"Well, I can see ADVANTAGES in this kind of barn, and I can see DISADVANTAGES."

"Let go of the nice doctor! . . . Shame on you . . . Let go of the . . ."

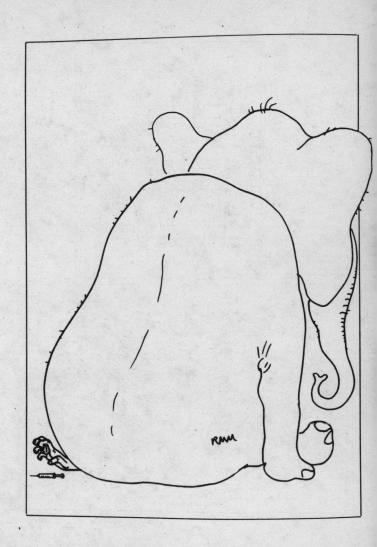

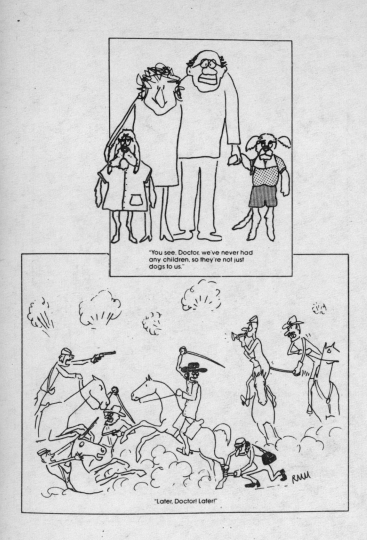

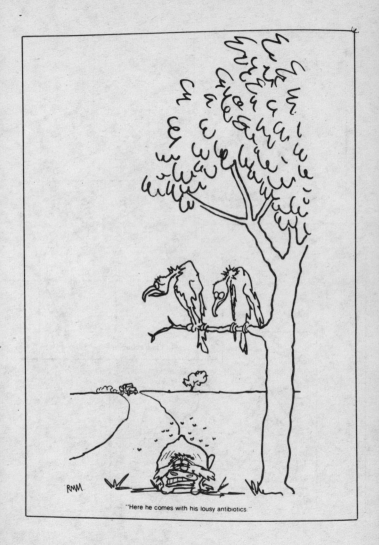

"Here he comes with his lousy antibiotics."

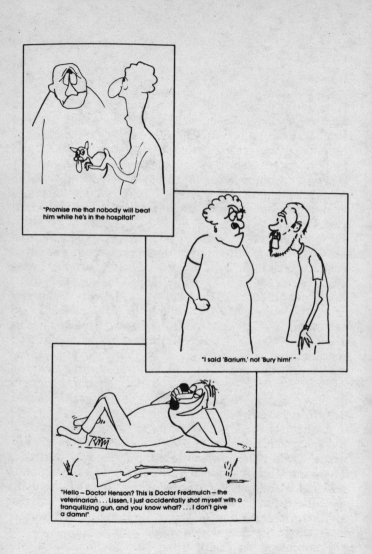

"Promise me that nobody will beat him while he's in the hospital!"

"I said 'Barium,' not 'Bury him!'"

"Hello — Doctor Henson? This is Doctor Fredmulch — the veterinarian . . . Lissen, I just accidentally shot myself with a tranquilizing gun, and you know what? . . . I don't give a damn!"

50

Chapter 9

I devoured sea stories as a kid. The whaling era particularly fascinated me. I read and re-read Moby Dick and every other book I could find about the days of the New England whalers. The names of New Bedford whaling ships became familiar to me, and my imagination was fired with images of Nantucket sleigh rides, great sperm whales breaching, the smoking try pots, and decks slippery with oil as whales were flensed and blubber cut up to be rendered into fuel for America's lamps. Of course, I outgrew this romantic infatuation, but nonetheless, my years at Pacific Ocean Park were special.

For three years before the park closed I cared for various sea mammals at this tourist attraction in Santa Monica. Pacific Ocean Park featured a sea circus and several staged animal acts. My patients would include trained dolphins, sea lions, harbour seals, a beluga (a dolphin commonly called the white whale), chimpanzees, an elephant, a dog act, and so on. The park was fifty miles from my practice in Thousand Oaks, so I accepted the responsibility on three conditions: that all visits would be in the evening, so my regular practice would not be interfered with; that my instructions would be followed (some wild-animal trainers ignore veterinarians' recommendations); and that I would be free to consult with other veterinarians.

At the time I was 'house doctor' at Pacific Ocean Park, a rival marine tourist attraction was featuring a trained pilot whale in its act. The owner of Pacific Ocean Park wanted a whale act. Thus it was that I was invited to go along on a series of whale-hunting expeditions. Although eventually we learned that the best way to capture a whale is to snare it as it plays near the bow of a boat, our initial thought was to incapacitate the animal with sedative drugs.

I purchased a tranquillizing rifle and modified the projectile syringes so that the needles had a harpoon barb on them. The first drug I decided to try was nicotine. An immobilizing solution was available from the company that manufactured the rifle and had been successfully used in a variety of wild and domestic species. This was prior to 1960 and none of the modern tranquillizing drugs were yet available for animal capture.

I had only been to the sea before on a troop ship, going to Europe and back a dozen years earlier. Now I found myself on a fishing boat, cruising the waters around the Channel Islands off the California coast. Several thousand pilot whale inhabit these waters, but they are not easily found.

For most of the first day I stayed on the bridge, eagerly watching for the pilot whales. I repeatedly thought that I saw them, but the more experienced crew identified what I saw as whitecaps, sea lions, driftwood, sharks, a manta ray, and sunfish.

By the second day, boredom had set in, and I retired below with a book. Then, from above, I heard our skipper, a professional whaler, sing out words that sent the adrenalin rushing through my veins.

'She blows! She blows! She blows!'

I rushed up on deck, and there they were, a school of two or three dozen pilot whales, gracefully arcing through the water off our bow, intermittently blowing. The skipper positioned himself on the bow platform, armed with a harpoon equipped with a small detachable head. Eventually a whale came within reach, and he harpooned it. The harpoon head detached, and as the whale dived, a line sounded. A float was attached to the end of the line, and it was pulled down into the depths by the sounding whale.

Our engines were cut and for about twenty minutes we drifted silently in the smooth water, peering in all directions for the whale to surface. It finally did so, about a quarter mile away, identifiable by the float it dragged. Engines started, and we pursued the animal which sounded again as we drew close.

'He'll only stay down about ten minutes this time,'

52

promised the skipper, 'but I don't think Doc will get a shot at her as long as he's in this boat. Doc, do you want to go out there alone in a skiff and keep quiet, and I think you'll have a chance at her?'

I agreed and went over the side into a small boat. The bigger vessel drew away from me, and suddenly I found myself completely alone, in an incredible silence, drifting somewhere over the whale, trying to see down into the dark waters. Off in the distance, in a great circle around me, the rest of the whale pod circled and blew. The tension was unbearable. I thought of the stories I had read as a boy, of whales coming up and splintering the waiting whale boats.

Finally the whale surfaced, only about fifty feet from me, and I fired, placing a dart just behind the dorsal fin. The whale dived at once, but it surfaced again in a couple of minutes and started swimming away from me. I started the skiff's motor and soon overtook the whale, picked up the float and pulled half the length of line into the skiff. Then the whale started to falter in its actions. I had injected it with only half the calculated immobilizing dose for its estimated weight because, of course, we didn't want it to drown. We just wanted to slow it down enough to enable us to net it. The main vessel was far away now, but I waved them in, knowing they were watching with binoculars.

The drugged whale was now desperately trying to stay afloat. Its movements were uncoordinated. It slowly towed me with the line, and the bigger boat could not seem to get closer to me.

It was then that I realized that the other whales had moved in close to us. They circled, on the surface, in obvious consternation. Our victim must have been sending out distress calls, and more and more whales of all sizes joined the small circle of concerned animals. I was suddenly aware of the great intelligence of these animals, of their involved social structure, of their ability to communicate. The excitement of the hunt and my eagerness to capture a live whale were replaced by a great wave of guilt at the anguish I had caused, of compassion for the concerned whales that, despite my presence, would not leave their disabled comrade. I was afraid, too; afraid that the whale would drown before the bigger boat could catch up with us, and afraid for my own safety. What if these gentle, harmless creatures decided to become vengeful? What chance would I have in that tiny boat if the whales responded to the threat to one of their members with human anger or with human vengeance? Above all, I was aware that what appeared to be simple fishlike creatures were thinking, emotional beings, capable of feeling fear and grief just as I could. I suddenly wanted that whale to be free.

The nicotine was wearing off. Coordination was returning, I cut the line. The orange float bobbed free, and there was a lump in my throat as the tired whale joined its circling mates. . .

Cetaceans – especially dolphins and whales – are wondrous creatures. I think I could easily have enjoyed a full-time career attending such patients. Their intelligence, cooperativeness, tolerance, and good nature were captivating.

Back when I was working with these creatures, beginning in 1959, little was known about cetacean medicine. The few veterinarians in the country treating sea mammals were in constant communication – the blind leading the blind. All of us were responsible for the health of valuable animals in marine amusement parks in California and Florida, and none of us really knew what we were doing. Yet, by applying our basic knowledge of medicine learned on other species, we were able to do a good job of caring for our unusual patients.

At Pacific Ocean Park, the ailments included eye injuries, nutritional deficiencies, skin infections, and other injuries. Dolphins sometimes swallow foreign bodies, so when one of them began to vomit persistently, he was taken, in an ambulance, on a stretcher to Thousand Oaks, where, for the first time in history, a barium gastro-intestinal series was performed on a sea mammal.

With dolphins it was customary to give intramuscular injections in the lumbar muscles. As a general rule, in most species, intramuscular injections are given in the massive hamstring muscles behind the thigh. Dolphins don't have legs, but they have an equivalent muscle group that propels the tail. It seemed logical to me that an intramuscular injection in a dolphin would be preferable if given in the huge muscles that propel the tail instead of in the much smaller loin muscles. Accordingly, the next time I had to give a penicillin injection to a dolphin I gave it in the hamstring area. It seemed a good idea to me. Penicillin has procaine in it. Procaine is a local anaesthetic and it is put in penicillin not to reduce the pain of injection, but to prolong the absorption of the drug. Unfortunately, I deposited the procaine penicillin close to a major nerve. As the nerve became anaesthetized the dolphin started to flounder. She had trouble staying afloat, and being an air breathing mammal, of course, my patient was in danger of drowning.

Into the shallow end of the dolphin pool I went and supported the squeaking, protesting animal. It was 8:30 p.m. I stayed in the water four and a half hours before the effects of the paralysing injection wore off and the dolphin could safely swim on her own. Obviously, I never again attempted an injection into the all important tail muscles.

Dolphins are forgiving creatures, and during the time I supported her in the waist deep water to keep her from drowning, a rapport developed between us. I told her how sorry I was that I had experimented on her, that my intentions had been sincere – to find a less painful injection site – and that I was going to stay with her until she recovered. The dolphin's fear of drowning seemed to abate. She relaxed and made a variety of sounds, but they did not have the ring of distress signals. Periodically she would see if her tail would function, and when it did, her joy was obvious.

As much as I enjoyed working with cetaceans I can't pretend I went from one touching experience to another.

Back in those days one veterinarian who used to call me

for advice on treating dolphins was a young Texan, Dr Sam Ridgway. This seems ironic today, because Sam is now one of the world's most knowledgeable authorities on cetacean medicine and the author of a distinguished book on the subject. Then a civilian, Sam had been employed by the US Navy, which was involved in research using trained dolphins, popularly called porpoises.

The naval research station was at Point Mugu, which is only about twenty-five miles from Thousand Oaks. When Sam went on vacation, he 'signed out' to me. The Navy personnel called me for advice a few times while Sam was gone, but I never had to make a visit. Except once, after Pacific Ocean Park had closed.

'Sam is out of town, and we have a problem,' the naval officer explained on the telephone. 'We are doing experiments with blindfolded porpoises. The blindfold consists of sort of a silicone rubber suction cup that fits over the eyes. Well, one of them came loose, and the porpoise swallowed it. Can you come over?'

'I'll be right there,' I answered. I jumped at the chance to treat a dolphin again, and besides, I was curious to see the Navy's somewhat mysterious facility.

At the naval base a sentry let my truck pass through the gates, and I proceeded to the waterfront. On a dock, next to a fenced lagoon, was a plastic portable swimming pool. It was the largest such pool I had ever seen, circular and wide but only about four-and-a-half feet deep. In it an Atlantic bottlenose dolphin, the familiar smiling grey performer, was casually swimming around the perimeter.

'Are you sure she swallowed the blindfold?' I asked.

'Absolutely,' the young officer responded. 'We saw her gulp it down. Sam says intestinal foreign bodies are a common cause of death in porpoises.'

'That's true,' I agreed, 'But it's only been an hour or two since it happened, and that thing is too big to leave her stomach. I believe that if I can make her vomit, it will come up.'

'Great!' said the officer. 'Make her vomit.'

Little was known about pharmacology as related to cetaceans. Those of us treating sea mammals learned by trial and error.

'Well,' I reasoned, 'if this were a dog, I'd give a dose of apomorphine to cause vomiting, so that's what I'll try.'

Searching in my small animal emergency bag, I found a vial of morphine tablets, but an empty apomorphine vial.

'Darn it,' I said. 'I'm sure apomorphine would serve as an emetic, but I don't know whether morphine would do the job.'

Actually, I knew nothing of the effects of either drug in this species. Apparently nobody else knew, either, because I had previously tried – unsuccessfully – to find this information.

I explained to the officer in charge. 'You see, in some species, such as the dog, morphine causes vomiting, followed by sedation and euphoria. In other species, such as the cat, morphine can cause wild excitement.'

'Well,' he replied, 'this porpoise retrieves balls and sticks. That's more like a dog than a cat, isn't it?'

'And she wags her tail, too!' offered one of the sailors.

These observations seemed logical. Besides, this was an emergency. Anyhow, I had always wanted to see the effects of morphine on a dolphin.

Four sailors in wet suits vaulted into the tank and gently held the porpoise while I gave the injection. I used the corresponding canine dose as a guide.

The men left the tank, and we all watched expectantly. For about ten minutes nothing happened. Then, almost imperceptibly at first, the animal began to swim more rapidly. She looped easily through the water, circling close to the sides of the tank. Periodically she blew, explosively exhaling and then almost simultaneously inhaling.

Soon it was apparent that the dolphin was blowing more frequently. She was swimming faster, no longer casually. There was a determination to her progress. A frothy wake emerged behind her. The blowing became more frequent, more forceful. The water began to slosh in the tank.

The dolphin was swimming ever faster. Instead of revealing just her blowhole and dorsal fin when she surfaced, she was arcing completely out of the water. She could easily have jumped out of the pool, but instead she held firmly to her circular course. Now her flukes were pounding the water, and she was attaining an amazing speed.

The plastic pool was swaying and rippling in response to the rhythmic waves created by the dolphin. The water was pouring over the sides. Sailors, civilian personnel, and a wet veterinarian braced their bodies against the sides of the pool. Faster and faster went the porpoise, a torpedo run amok.

'The tank's going to go!' yelled a man.

'Stop her!' shouted the officer. 'Get in there and stop her!'

Instantly the four sailors in wet suits vaulted back into the pool. They grabbed futilely at the gleaming grey body as it sped past them.

'Back me!' hollered a big, husky, young frogman. He stepped into the path of the madly churning porpoise. The other men leaped into line behind him. I gasped in disbelief. The beak of a dolphin at full speed is a formidable weapon, capable of stunning a large shark. The sailor caught this beak in the crook of his arm, as he would have caught a football. The line of men reeled backwards, but they kept their feet and stopped the animal. She was transferred to a stretcher, and there she quivered and vibrated and squeaked and puffed – but she did not vomit.

'I need some Nalline,' I told the officer desperately.

'What's that?'

'It's an antidote for morphine. Quick! Get me to the base hospital!'

I was rushed in a Jeep to the infirmary. I ran into the reception area, sloshing about in soaking wet coveralls, followed by three men clad in rubber wet suits. A gaping young physician soon stood shaking his head, trying to comprehend my story.

'This is urgent!' I pleaded. 'I'm a veterinarian. We have an adverse reaction to morphine in a porpoise. I need Nalline in a hurry!'

'A porpoise?' the doctor sputtered. 'Out there? In the ocean? You gave morphine? Why? To make her vomit? To make a porpoise vomit?'

One of the sailors offered to help. 'Yes! She swallowed her blindfold. It's about this big and made of rubber. It looks like a falsie. It's in her stomach!'

'A falsie?' said the bewildered physician, looking from me to the dripping frogman.

By the time the situation was understood, and I had signed numerous documents in order to procure the Nalline, the effects of the morphine had worn off. The dolphin was blissfully cruising her pool again.

Sam phoned me two weeks later.

'You know,' he said, 'that piece of silocone rubber is still in that porpoise's stomach. I X-rayed her, and I can see it plain as day.'

'How about fishing it out through a gastroscope?' I suggested. 'You could borrow one from the base hospital.'

'I don't know how we stand with them,' Sam mused. 'They're still talking about the frogmen and all that stuff. Kind of shook 'em up, I guess.'

'I'm sure sorry about that!' I said.

'Oh, hell! I'm not!' said Sam. 'I've always wondered what morphine would do to a porpoise!'

Chapter 10

For the first couple of years my practice was limited to house calls. This was the accepted thing for livestock and horses, but it was not customary for the treatment of small animals. My station wagon was my office, and between it and my doctor's bag, I carried most of what I needed for dogs and cats.

Surgery was a more challenging problem. Weather permitting, I used the tail gate of my station wagon for an operating table, but most of the time I used an ironing board in the owner's house.

Elaborate surgical procedures were usually referred to animal hospitals in the city, but I was able to do most routine procedures on the ironing boards.

Jappy was a sweet, little, black mixed spaniel with an undershot jaw and a perpetually wagging tail. Her little tail would gyrate so vigorously when she was spoken to that it seemed to disengage her hind end from her front end so that, while her front end walked towards one, the hind end would wobble from side to side and seemed to have difficulty keeping up with her front half.

Jappy's owners were a delightful retired couple in their sixties, Emil and Helen Klein. They made an appointment for me to spay Jappy in their home. I anaesthetized the happy two-year-old little spaniel and positioned her on the ironing board. As I clipped the hair from her belly with electric clippers, I noticed that Jappy was in heat.

'Yes,' said Mrs Klein, 'we procrastinated and put this thing off until it was too late. Is that a problem? Can she still be spayed?'

'Well,' I responded, 'yes, she can, but the reproductive organs are greatly enlarged during oestrus, and we'll have to be very careful. It is riskier to do it at this time, but she's anaesthetized, and I'm all set to go, so let's get on with it.'

Several minutes later I wished that I had postponed the

surgery. As I attempted to exteriorize the right ovary so that I could tie it off, Jappy's ovarian artery ruptured, and in moments I had a belly full of blood.

The Kleins sat smiling benevolently at me from across the room. I was glad they could not see my face, concealed by an operating mask. I said nothing, but agonized silently as I sponged, mopped, extended my incision, and hunted for the bleeding stump. Ah! at long last I recovered it, stopped the haemorrhage with artery forceps, and then gratefully and carefully ligated the stump.

'My goodness,' said Mrs. Klein. 'I had no idea there'd be so much blood. This is really a major operation, isn't it?'

Mrs Klein was right. A spay is most certainly a major piece of abdominal surgery, and if veterinarians are complacent about this operation, it is because they do it so often. Yet, when something goes amiss, as it did with Jappy, it becomes obvious just how major an operation a spay is.

Jappy recovered nicely from her ironing-board pan-hysterectomy and lived to be fifteen years of age.

After making hundreds of house calls on small animals and after doing dozens of operations on ironing boards, I was happy when the day came that I could open an office in Thousand Oaks. At about the same time I got myself an honest-to-goodness small-animal hospital, however modest it was, I got to thinking it would be nice to have better equipment for my large-animal practice as well.

Most veterinarians engaged in large-animal practice used automobiles to make their rounds when I graduated from professional school in 1956. During the next decade, however, the mobile veterinary unit, manufactured by several different companies, came into existence. Today the great majority of American practitioners use these units. They are usually constructed of white fibreglass, fit into the bed of a pickup truck, and they are conveniently equipped with running water, an electric refrigerator, and compartments for the astounding variety of equipment the large-animal practitioner must carry, including many drugs, ropes, farrier tools, huge dental instruments, devices to pull calves during difficult deliveries, and so on. As soon as I was able to, I gave up the station wagon I had been using as a practice vehicle and bought a mobile unit. It was the first one west of the Mississippi, and my clients' eyes bugged out when they saw my sink, with hot and cold running water, my oxygen tank, and all of the other gadgets the unit was equipped with.

'Looks like an ice-cream truck,' said many of the people I called upon. Indeed, one day as I searched a suburban neighbourhood for a house at which a sick pony awaited me, the driver of an ice-cream truck glared at me, hands on her hips, lower jaw jutting out, scowling. She thought I had invaded her territory.

Allen Carling-Smith was a rancher. He had a fine herd of polled Hereford cattle in Hidden Valley, and I was often at the ranch several times a week. Although most of my clients eventually accepted my 'ice-cream truck,' Allen invariably greeted me with 'I'll have two strawberry popsicles, please.' This went on for months. Finally, I put some popsicles in the freezer compartment of the refrigerator in the unit, and the next time Allen asked me for popsicles, I got out of the pickup cab, opened the refrigerator compartment, and presented him with a strawberry, a lemon, and an orange. Then I added fifteen cents to the ranch's bill that month and itemized the charge 'For popsicles.'

The years have wrought changes. Mobile veterinary units are so commonplace in the rural American scene that nobody makes remarks any longer about their looking like ice-cream trucks. You can't buy a popsicle for a nickel any longer, either.

Chapter 11

'This is Keller's Jungle Killers. Can you come as quickly as possible, please?' the voice on the telephone pleaded. 'Our entire cat act has been poisoned.'

Keller's Jungle Killers was a circus act. Big cats of various species were all trained to perform together. I could tell from the urgency in the caller's voice that something terrible had happened, and I hurried to my vehicle, started the engine, and headed towards Agoura. The Keller Ranch was located in Triunfo Canyon, deep in the Santa Monica mountains, the coastal range that separates us from the Pacific Ocean.

In those days, when horses or livestock died, the wild animals in our area were often fed the butchered meat, providing, of course, that the cause of death would not endanger the animals consuming the meat. Jungleland, for example, provided a cost-free service and picked up dead stock from all over southern California. Most of the meat was fed to the scores of big cats in our community, and to other carnivorous species. Veterinarians in our area knew this so, when a large animal had to be destroyed for humane reasons, we always asked the owner how the carcass was going to be disposed of. If we were told that Jungleland was going to pick it up, we explained to the owner that since the meat was going to be consumed by lions and tigers and such, we could not destroy the animal in the usual manner, by quickly administering an intravenous barbiturate anaesthetic. To do so would mean that the carcass would be toxic and unsafe for consumption. Instead the animal in question had to be destroyed with a gunshot into the brain. The meat, after butchering, was then perfectly safe for the big cats to eat.

Every few years a mistake would occur. Perhaps a veterinarian new to our area and unaware of the victim's ultimate destination would be involved. He would administer the lethal dose of barbiturate to the horse or cow in question and not know that the owner would dispose of the carcass by calling Jungleland.

Or, perhaps the owner would be at fault, telling the veterinarian that they wanted an anaesthetic to be given and that the carcass was going to be buried or be taken to a rendering plant. Later, after the animal was dead and the veterinarian had left the premises, the owner would reconsider after learning the cost of having the carcass hauled away by a stock hauling service. He would then call Jungleland, and not revealing the cause of death, simply say that they had a dead animal they wanted removed free of charge.

In this manner, an occasional toxic carcass would be butchered and fed to the big cats. This apparently is what happened to Keller's Jungle Killers.

When I arrived at the Keller Ranch, I found a group of people – owners, trainers, and neighbours – in a state of consternation. The Keller act consisted of a mixed group of ten big cats. A tiger, a black panther, two lions, a leopard, and a puma were showing signs of severe intoxication ranging from loss of balance to coma. Four other cats, a tiger, two more pumas, and a jaguar, were less severely affected, displaying only mild signs of intoxication. The family dog, a malemute named 'Hexy,' had eaten some of the meat and was also showing signs of intoxication.

It took several hours to examine all of the animals and begin treatment on those requiring medication. Most severely affected was a Bengal tiger, a magnificent specimen weighing several hundred pounds. He was in a coma, devoid of all reflexes, taking only an occasional breath, and I feared for his survival.

A neighbour, a young woman who was a registered nurse, volunteered to stay up all night with the tiger. I catheterized a vein, hooked it up to intravenous fluids, and left instructions to keep the tiger warm and to turn him every half hour to prevent congestion of his lungs. I also started antibiotics to prevent pneumonia, which I knew from previous experience was a common complication in cases of this kind. The largest of the big cats detoxify barbiturates very, very slowly, and I knew that this tiger would not regain consciousness for many days, if he survived at all.

The black panther was also severely affected, and I was concerned for his survival too.

By the second day I knew that all of the animals, with the possible exception of the tiger, were going to make it. He was still in a deep coma and being fed intravenously, but I saw no signs of consciousness returning. Even if he did survive, I worried that permanent brain damage would result.

The nurse volunteered to spend a second night in the tiger's cage, but by this time a shift of volunteers had been organized to stay beside the comatose beast. All of the volunteers expressed concern that the tiger might suddenly regain consciousness while they were in the cage. I knew that this was not possible, but I sympathized with their apprehension. A few months earlier I attempted to take the rectal temperature of one of the other tigers, a much smaller individual. He was confined to a squeeze cage and protested mightily when examined, but to no avail, because he was compressed by the moveable side walls of the squeeze cage. I could not quite reach his tail, so I suggested that he be manoeuvred backwards by placing a board in front of him. A two-by-four-inch plank was put into place in front of his chest, and when I lifted his tail to insert the thermometer, he bit the board in half. The power in those jaws is fearsome.

Eventually, the Bengal tiger recovered, but not for two weeks during which time he did develop pneumonia.

With intensive care, massive doses of chloramphenical (an antibiotic), and constant supervision, he recuperated. In a month he was back in the act.

The black panther recovered more quickly, and a year later showed his gratitude by sinking his teeth into my forearm. I still have the scars.

*   *   *

Indeed, having a practice that includes circus acts and wild animals has prevented my life from becoming humdrum. In fact, the John Strong Circus was headquartered right behind our veterinary clinic. Stand at the back door and you could see the gaily painted circus wagons and their tethered Indian elephant.

John Strong had collected a variety of animal 'freaks' that were part of his show, and some of the calls I received were, to say the least, unusual.

For example, one day I was presented with a six-legged sheep with a broken leg. The case card reads, 'Fractured metacarpus of the right middle leg.'

I wonder if any other veterinarian in the world has ever been called to see a two-headed calf with bloat. The Strongs had a healthy calf, about nine months of age, with two heads. The two heads were united at the skull, the muzzles were complete and separate, and the two skulls shared a single central eye. Thus there were three eyes, and as far as I could determine, all three eyes had normal vision. Now, this calf was bloated, and the owner was understandably concerned. A two-headed calf is not easily replaced.

The usual way of treating bloat is to pass a stomach tube in order to allow the gas to escape and to permit the administration of medication. The problem was, I didn't know which head to treat. I asked John if the calf ate with both mouths. 'No,' he answered, 'only the one on the left, but when he chews, both heads chew even though the food is only in the left mouth.' Accordingly, I passed the tube through the mouth in the left head and successfully reduced the bloat.

Because of the popularity of leg of lamb and pickled calftongue, I asked Mr Strong if he had considered breeding his unusual animals. 'I've got an even better idea, Doc,' he said. 'I have a four-legged rooster I'd like to sell to Colonel Sanders.'

Chapter 12

I am not afraid of animals. If I were I would not have selected veterinary medicine as a career, and I certainly would not have elected to treat such a wide variety of species. However, within many species there have been individuals that I learned to fear because they were particularly aggressive or treacherous. These were not only animals of the exotic species, but dogs, cats, horses, and cattle as well.

I recall a particularly nasty merino ram. To his owner's delight, this ram had charged and mauled several people who made the mistake of trespassing in his pasture. The owner referred to the ram as his 'watch buck.' The animal not only protected his own property, but on one occasion battered his way into a neighbour's kitchen and ran the family out.

I am not afraid of sheep in general, but I was afraid of this ram. He once ran me up a fence and still managed to mash my ankle against a post. Happily, he finally knocked his master down and butted and mauled him about in the mud and manure. Shortly afterward, I was called to castrate the ram, a task I gleefully performed.

Working with exotic species, as I do, calls for a bit of extra caution. Again, I like these animals and they do not ordinarily frighten me. There is an exception. There is one kind of animal I uniformly fear. I am afraid of chimpanzees.

Young chimps are no problem. They are fun and bright and manageable. Mature chimps are another matter. I am terrified of mature chimpanzees, particularly males.

I enjoy stepping up to an elephant, lion, or even a gorilla, but I have to steel myself to examine a big chimp. I try not to show my fear. I act confident, laugh a lot, and casually pat their low, thick craniums. I look into their faces and pretend not to be intimidated by their great white fangs and shifty, brown humanoid eyes that gleam with cunning and treachery.

Chimps have the mind of a diabolical human being – a homicidal maniac with the IQ of a four-year-old child and the strength of a Russian weightlifter. I tremble as they take my puny hand in their enormous mitts. As they lovingly hug me, encircling my torso with their great hairy, sinewy arms, I know the revulsion a 'frigid' wife must feel when approached by a loutish husband.

Once, I liked chimpanzees. I treated many of them in my early practice years, but they were all little fellows. I enjoyed them as patients. Then, one day, an animal trainer asked me to treat his five-year-old male. After I readily agreed to do so, the trainer warned me, 'This is a mature male, Doctor, and he's kind of rough.' I assured him that I had treated chimps before and was not worried.

This chimp, a circus performer, was kept, with others in his act, in a long, narrow room. One wall was lined with cages, each containing a hooting, pounding ape. The chimp I was to examine weighed eighty-five pounds – not a particularly large individual, but his wrists and arms were thicker than the trainer's.

I completed my examination uneventfully and then announced that I wanted to give the animal an injection. The trainer inserted his thumb into the chimp's mouth and holding him by the lower jaw put his own nose right up to the chimp's face. 'The doctor's gonna give you a shot,' he explained to the chimp, 'and if you move, I'll tear your [obscenity deleted] head off. If you bite me, I'll kill you!' promised the trainer.

Then, an assistant, another animal trainer, got behind the chimp, took a full nelson wrestling hold on the animal and grunted, 'Go ahead and shoot him, Doc!'

I was somewhat annoyed by all these precautions and by what I felt was an unnecessary display of threats and force. 'Look,' I said, 'there's nothing to this. I'm going to give him an injection in his hind end. He won't even feel it!'

I was standing behind the assistant trainer who, with his

back to me, was obscuring the chimp he held in the wrestling hold. That chimpanzee must have understood my words because he immediately reached back with his foot and grabbed me by the ankle.

'Go ahead, Doc! Shoot him!'

'I can't. His foot's got my foot!'

I was surprised by the strength in the prehensile foot. My ankle felt as if it were being compressed by a steel band. I could not free it, so I used my other foot to kick at the chimp's leg. I thought I could kick his foot from my ankle. Instead, his other foot shot back, grabbed my free ankle, and with a sharp pull he jerked me off my feet. Now I was sitting on the floor, the last in line. First came the trainer, holding the chimp by the lower jaw; then there was the chimp; then the assistant, holding the chimp with a full nelson; and finally there I was, sitting, both ankles grasped in a death-grip by the chimp's feet.

At this point, I was embarrassed but still not afraid. In fact, I was laughing at the ludicrous situation.

'He's got me,' I told the trainers, 'but here's where I get him!' I jabbed the needle into the chimp's thigh and quickly injected him.

An explosion followed. Screaming, but amazingly never biting the trainer's thumbs in his mouth, the chimp wrenched free from the trainer. The assistant, still holding the chimp, fell over on his back, the chimp on top of him. I pulled my ankles free and scooted backward along the floor. The chimp reached both arms out toward me, clutching and raging.

I backed away in alarm. The only door to the room was blocked by the chimp and the two struggling men who now had the animal on the floor. The trainer weighed 155 pounds, the assistant, nearly 200. I was amazed to see the 85-pound animal alternately flipping those men off the floor. The strength in those arms was inconceivable. I must have blanched as I realized that he paid no attention to his captors. He was looking at me and raging at me. He wanted *me*.

'Don't turn him loose,' I suggested.

'We're trying', Doc! We're tryin!'

After several exhausting minutes the two men worked the screaming animal back to its cage.

'Can I help?' I asked. Why waste all the adrenalin coursing through my blood vessels?

'No! Stay back. If you come close, you'll just make him worse! He wants you!'

I did not come close. Like a maiden being saved from a fate worse than death by two heroic knights, I cringed anxiously against the far wall.

At last the chimp had been pushed back into his cage – all but his right arm. As the trainers leaned against the cage door, that arm reached out towards me. The hand grasped and clawed in my direction.

When the cage door was finally forced closed and latched, the chimp stopped howling and simply glared at me malevolently, holding the bars in his mighty fingers and rattling them fiercely.

'Whew!' Both men wiped the sweat from their brows and necks. I sidled past them and gladly made my exit.

'I told you he was rough, Doctor,' the trainer said.

'Tex,' I answered, 'the thing that shakes me up is that he never attempted to injure either one of you. He acted as if he were in an uncontrollable fury, yet he was able to confine his anger and direct it all at me. Was it an act? I know that primates will indulge in an intimidation display to frighten an intruder. If he had got loose and come after me, do you think he would have backed off if I'd stood my ground?'

'Doctor Miller,' the trainer said solemnly, 'if we had turned loose of that animal, he would have torn your face away from your skull in a few seconds.'

I have been afraid of chimpanzees ever since.

Chimp trainers tell me they must completely dominate their charges in order to control them. Unless a chimp regards its trainer with trust, respect, and fear (if it misbehaves), the trainer soon loses control. For that

70

reason, many trained chimps are retired as they reach maturity and start to assert themselves, particularly if they are males.

Not only are chimps frightening, I believe that they can hatch plots.

When I was the veterinarian for Pacific Ocean Park, the park featured a variety show that included a chimp act. Three young chimps, dressed in adorable little suits, put on a show that delighted the audience. One of the chimps did a wire-walking routine. Midway across the cable, the chimp would look down at the audience, shake its hands and scream in mock anguish. Children loved this act. What the audience did not know was that beneath the grandstand was a man with an air-rifle aimed at the chimp. The rifle inspired the chimp to complete the trip across the cable.

After the chimp routine, a special guest act performed the grand finale. One summer this act consisted of three divers from Acapulco. They ascended a one-hundred-foot tower (which was actually eighty feet high) and did breathtaking dives into a water tank. One night, as usual after finishing their act, the chimps left the stage as the three divers ran on, resplendent in scarlet capes. When the two groups passed in the wings, each chimp, as if on a pre-arranged signal, attacked one of the men. Before the animals could be restrained, each of the men had suffered severe bite wounds. These were young chimps, but this incident illustrates the kind of behaviour of which these animals are capable.

Sometimes in dealing with a chimp, finesse, not force, is required. We should be able to outsmart a chimp, shouldn't we?

Jim Bedford owned a trained chimpanzee named Jerry. Jerry was a performer, but he had a problem. He suffered from stage fright and would develop severe diarrhoea as soon as he began his act. Jim, the owner, consulted me, and after examining Jerry and running some diagnostic tests, I concluded that the problem was entirely psychological. I prescribed Metropectin® tablets, to be given prior to a

71

performance. This product contains kaolin and pectin which help to solidify and harden the stool, plus an anticholinergic drug which slows down the action of the bowel. Anticholinergic drugs, however, have side effects. They tend to cause blurred vision, sensitivity to bright light, and dryness of the mouth.

The owner assured me that the chimp was extremely suspicious and would refuse any oral medication, regardless of flavouring. The tablets in question have a somewhat chalky, lemony taste. Since chimps are extremely intelligent and cunning, it is no small task to outwit them, but I decided to attempt it with Jerry.

I showed up one day at Jerry's home, wearing street clothes and carrying a white paper bag filled with a thousand Metropectin tablets. The owner greeted me, and followed by the chimp, we went out on the lawn to talk.

'How have you been, Jim?' I asked, dipping into the bag and munching a tablet. 'Want some candy?'

'Thanks,' said Jim, taking a handful. Jerry at this point started hooting, grimacing, and shaking his hands.

'What does he want?' I asked.

'I think he wants some candy,' Jim answered.

'May he have some?' I asked, crunching down on another tablet. Jerry shrieked his approval and started wildly bouncing up and down at this.

'Not unless he earns it,' said Jim with his mouth full.

'Jerry, make a somersault. Good boy! Jerry, applaud! Do a handstand! Walk on your hands! Jerry, climb the tree. Giant swings, Jerry! Swing like a monkey! Good boy! Now take a bow! Throw a kiss! OK, here's a candy.'

Jerry popped the pill into his mouth delightedly. As long as I live, I shall never forget the look on his face. His expression clouded. He pulled his lower lip down like a flap, extracted the tablet, studied it suspiciously, stuck his tongue out disgustedly and finally squinted at us sideways. Jim and I ignored him and munched another tablet. Finally, Jerry put the pill back into his mouth and thoughtfully crunched it down, then – triumph – without too much enthusiasm he started to hoot and beg for another tablet.

That was the end of Jerry's problem, but his master didn't fare as well. I saw him a week later.

'How are you, Jim?'

'Not too good,' he answered. 'I've been awfully consti-pated, the light bothers my eyes, and my mouth's terribly dry. Been sittin' in the bathroom all week with the lights out, drinking like a fish. But Jerry is fine! He always takes his medicine, just so long as I take some first!'

Chimps and medication – especially injections – have often been a risky mix. After my earlier experience, I was forced to learn some tricks.

I recall one big, mean male that was delivered to the clinic in a van. The trainer told me that if I attempted to inject this animal myself it would cost me my life. In order to tranquillize the chimp for examination, I loaded a syringe, then handed it to the trainer. The trainer then gave the syringe to the chimp, who, on command, gave himself the injection. Several times during subsequent visits the chimp injected itself in my presence.

Then there were the two older chimps, a male and a female, that shared a cage at Jungleland. These animals were used for exhibition only. They were not trained and could not be handled. The male suffered a dental abscess. I offered him a banana, and when he reached through the bars for it, I quickly injected phencyclidine into his wrist. Raging, he jerked his hand into the cage, pounded the floor and raced in circles. But in a few minutes the drug took effect, and the chimp slept peacefully while I extracted a molar.

Many months later, the female needed treatment. With syringe in right hand and banana in left, I attempted to lure her to the bars. But the male, remembering my treachery, seized her by the arm and tried to keep her from me. She resisted him, loudly insisting that she knew what she was doing. In a most human manner he pleaded and threatened. Vehemently espousing woman's liberation,

73

the female broke away from the male and reached out for the banana. As I jabbed the syringe into her arm, the male slapped his forehead with both hands, looked up at the sky, and seemed to cry, 'I told you so!'

The most grotesque experience I ever had with a chimpanzee makes a story I hesitate to relate because it sounds fictional. Yet, it happened.

My telephone rang at one o'clock in the morning. A man with a foreign accent told me that several other veterinarians had advised him to call me. The man was calling on behalf of his wife, a member of an Arabic royal family, whom, for the purpose of anonymity, I shall call Princess Fatima. It seems that the princess owned a five-year-old pet female chimpanzee she had obtained when the animal was a baby.

This chimp lived in a large cage in the back yard, but was allowed out during the day to eat with the family. She sat in a highchair at meal times and used silverware and a napkin. She also was allowed to vacuum clean the house and mow the lawn with a power mower.

During the past year, the chimp had escaped from her cage several times. Using her own rule book, she refused to return to her cage on these occasions. She had, in fact, gone on a spree of vandalism. The morning before I was called, the chimp had escaped again and had gone on a rampage. Neither the princess nor her husband could regain control of the screaming, somersaulting miscreant. The princess then called her first husband, who, it seems, had visiting rights with the chimp.

The first husband, as a concerned and responsible parent should, soon appeared. He scolded the wayward chimp while attempting to drag her back to the cage with a length of chain fastened around her neck. This chimp had never before injured a human, but she savagely attacked her 'father,' lacerating his hand so severely that hospitalization and the services of a surgical specialist were required.

The unexpected attack totally unnerved the princess and her current consort. They passed the end of the chain

74

through a fence, and with the chimp at the opposite end of the chain, the princess had been holding on for eight hours! Meanwhile, her husband had been unsuccessfully telephoning for help. He had called the humane society, the police, the fire department, the zoo, his family physician, a psychiatrist, and more than sixty veterinarians. Nobody offered to help him, but several veterinarians told him of a Doctor Miller in Thousand Oaks who loved chimps and who owned a tranquillizing gun.

I wondered if a colleague was playing a practical joke on me, but the poor man's desperation convinced me of his sincerity. 'Plez come!' he begged. 'Poor woman is nirly exhosted! Hendz oll blistered! Plez come help os! We pay whatever you say!'

'Why don't you wire the chain to the fence?' I asked. 'So the princess can let go.'

'Oh, Doctor,' he cried joyously. 'Already you help os!'

Having brilliantly solved the problem of the owner's blistered hands, I somewhat apprehensively agreed to make an emergency call at their home which was about seventy miles away, in a luxurious beach-front suburb of Los Angeles.

I arrived at their magnificent marina home at about 2:30 a.m. A thin, dark-moustachioed man and Princess Fatima met me in front of the house. The princess was about five feet tall and of similar girth – a little, round, brown woman dressed in a harem-style diaphanous lounging suit with – yes – slippers with upturned toes. Unlimbering my Cap-Chur® gun, I felt like a hero out of *The Arabian Nights*.

'Where is the chimp?' I asked.

'In the back, Doctor,' they chorused. The yard was surrounded by a solid, six-foot, wooden fence. The couple were so terrified of their former pet that they would not allow me to open the gate. 'What if she has got loose?' they cried. 'Be careful, Doctor!'

I chinned-up on the fence and looked upon an expansive yard. Most of it was landscaped in lawn and garden. In one corner was the chimp's cage. A ten-foot-square wooden affair with a front of half-inch steel mesh. One corner of the cage had been prised loose by the chimp when it escaped. Closer to the house I saw a swimming pool in the patio, well illuminated with spotlights. A four-foot-high chain-link fence surrounded the pool. Attached to the fence with a chain was the chimpanzee curled up in a motionless ball.

I opened the gate and approached the chimp, followed by the fearful owners who kept urging me to be careful. Nearing the animal, I heard rhythmic snoring. The chimp did not respond to my voice. Finally, I touched her. She snored on, in deep sleep.

'Did you give her anything?' I asked.

They had. It seems that, before they were able to contact me, the owners had called their physician and asked if they could give the chimp some of the princess's sleeping medicine. The doctor had suggested a tablespoon, and while the princess was holding the chain through the fence, her husband had offered the chimp a spoonful of medication. The chimp shot its fingers through the fence, grabbed the bottle, and drained it.

Putting aside my gun, I read the label on the two-ounce medicine bottle. It listed a physician's name. It was a Chinese name – something like Yang-soo, M.D.

I phoned the pharmacy. No answer. I called Dr Yang-soo. He sleepily answered the phone, and I apologetically explained the problem, knowing that he had already suffered other chimp calls during the night. 'She drank *all* the medicine,' I said. 'Ooooh, you got tlouble!' the doctor answered. 'Big tlouble!'

'What was in the bottle?' I asked anxiously.

'Eriksasecunura!' he responded in his native accent.

'I beg your pardon?'

'Eriksasecunura! Eriksasecunura!'

'What is that,' I asked, 'a herb?'

'No,' he said in exasperation. 'Barbitulate!'

Aha. A flash! 'Elixir of seconal?'

'Yes! Yes!' said the doctor.

I thanked him and apologized for disturbing his sleep.

Then I gave the chimp antibiotics to help prevent pneumonia, injected caffeine, and left additional caffeine injections and instructions to keep the chimp warm and to turn her hourly. It was now past 3:00 a.m. I suggested that if the chimp was not awake by noon, she would probably require hospitalization and intravenous fluids. The owners gratefully paid me for my time, and we had a morning cup of coffee together.

I called that evening and was pleased to hear that the chimp was fully awake and seemed quite normal. The princess asked if I could find a new home for her pet, preferably with a theatrical act or with a circus.

'She has been brought up like a human child,' she explained, 'and I cannot bear the thought of her spending her life in a zoo. She knows so many things and is so responsive. But I cannot keep her any longer and risk somebody else being injured.'

I gave the princess the names of several persons who used trained chimpanzees. At the head of the list was a motion picture animal ranch that employed a young resident veterinarian, Dr Martin Dinnes, who later became one of the nation's foremost specialists in wild and zoo animals.

Two days later the princess called to thank me for my help and tell me that Dr Dinnes had accepted her chimp.

About five years passed. Then, at a veterinary convention, a group of wild-animal practitioners sat around the hotel swimming pool swapping tales of the outrageous incidents this kind of practice generates. Marty Dinnes told how a hippopotamus had escaped from his compound, and how he had run the animal down on horseback, brandishing a tranquillizing pistol. When the laughter subsided, he said, 'Bob, tell them about the chimp.'

I related the entire story, and when I had finished, Marty asked, 'Did I ever tell you what happened the next day?'

'I heard you accepted the chimp, came out and tranquillized it, and took it home in your car,' I responded.

'Well,' said Dr Dinnes, 'It wasn't that simple. I came out, and there she was, awake, in that cage with the half-inch

77

steel wire-mesh front. I couldn't get the barrel of my Cap-Chur gun through the mesh, so I knocked out a knot in the wooden portion of the cage. Through the knothole, I was able to aim and fire a dart into her hind end.'

'That was smart,' I complimented him.

'Oh?' he retorted. 'As soon as the dart hit that chimp, she instantly pulled it out, whirled around and threw the dart back through the knothole! I nearly lost an eye! The needle embedded itself in the bone right under the orbit,' he said, pointing to a small round scar under his eye.

That is the incredible ending to an incredible tale, but it illustrates why I fear the chimpanzee, an animal possessed of great strength, a frightening temper, and sinister cunning.

Chapter 13

Weekends are busy in our practice. People are using their horses, so many injuries occur. Horses often get colic on weekends, I suspect because their usual feeding schedule is disrupted. The owners may sleep late on Saturday morning, so the horse is fed late. Then, on Saturday evening, the veterinarian is needed to treat a horse with colic.

My calls were completed one Saturday night. I drove home, parked my truck, and silently prayed for a quiet evening. At ten o'clock I was comfortably watching television with my family when the telephone rang.

'This is Bob Nesbitt,' said a voice with an Oklahoma

78

accent. 'You don't know me but my place is in Box Canyon, and I've got a bloated bull here I'm worried about.'

Box Canyon is nearly thirty miles from my home.

'Do you want me to see him, or to tell you what to do?' I asked. Nearly all veterinarians serve as free information centres. For every animal we actually see, we probably advise and prescribe for several more. This is not an ideal situation, but it is the way things are.

'Well, can you tell me what to do?'

'How badly is he bloated? Is he down?'

'No! He's up and he's eating, but his belly is blown up on the left side, and he's a good bull and I'm worried 'bout him.'

'Okay,' I said. With his southwestern drawl, the caller sounded like a cowman, and I thought that he would be capable of following my instructions.

'First of all, don't let him eat anymore. What did he bloat on?'

'Alfalfa.'

'Okay! Don't let him eat. Pass a stomach tube down into his stomach and see if that will let some of the gas off.'

Bloat is a common affliction in cattle, and our first approach is usually to pass a tube down into the rumen. In order to do this, we hold the mouth open with a speculum, or gag. A block of wood with a hole in it serves admirably for this purpose. All experienced cattlemen are familiar with this procedure.

'That's the trouble, Doc!' he said. 'Ain't got a tube.'

'Well, you can make one from a length of garden hose,' I suggested. 'Just cut off seven or eight feet and round the cut edge so it won't injure him when you pass it down.'

'Hey, Doc. Why didn't I think of that? Thank you for the advice.'

'After the gas comes out,' I said, 'pour an ounce or two of turpentine down through the tube. It will help prevent further gas formation.'

'Thank you, Doc. I'll do that. Much obliged!'

'If that doesn't help, you let me know.'

'Sure will, Doc. Thank you, kindly.'

Sunday morning was quiet. I got up early and fed my horses. After breakfast the telephone rang. It was Mr Nesbitt.

'Doc, I just wanted to thank you for all your help last night. Mighty nice of you.'

'You're welcome. How is the bull?'

'Oh, he's just fine! Passed the hose and the gas come up, and we give him the turpentine and he's happy as a clam out there grazin'.'

'That's fine,' I said. 'I'm glad I could be of service, and I appreciate your calling to tell me how it came out.'

'You bet, Doc. Now, tell me, how are we going to get the tube out?'

'What?' I said, startled.

'The hose? How are we going to get it out?'

'What do you mean?' I asked. 'How can he be grazing if the tube is still in him? Didn't you pull it back out? You're not supposed to leave it in him.'

'Oh, we figured that, but afore we could get it out, he bit it off and swallered it.'

'He what?'

'Yup! Swallered four foot of it. We cut it seven foot long, and we only got three foot left.'

'Didn't you use a speculum? Didn't you put something in his mouth so he couldn't bite the hose?'

'Doc, you never said nothing about that. Me and my brother-in-law just cut off seven foot of hose, stuck it down him, and he bit off and swallered four foot.'

'That's going to cause serious problems,' I said. 'That length of hose has to be removed. It will take a surgical operation.'

'Well, then,' Nesbitt said, 'come on out, and we'll do 'er.'

As I drove into Box Canyon, I was glad it was Sunday. That meant that, barring emergencies, I had plenty of time to do a rumenotomy on the bull. This operation is done with the animal standing, under regional anaesthesia. We open the left side, expose the rumen, the largest of the four bovine stomach chambers, sew the rumen to the skin, and then incise the rumen, creating a window directly into the stomach. I had done many rumenotomies to recover wire and nails that had penetrated the stomach wall. 'Hardware' operations, we called them. Nowadays, magnets placed in the bovine stomach hold the various bits of metal that cattle eat, and 'Hardware Disease' is less common than when I started practice. I did a rumenotomy on a bison once, to remove a copy of the *Los Angeles Times*. The massive Sunday edition caused a near fatal impaction of the rumen. I had never performed the operation for the removal of a garden hose, however. This was going to be a new experience.

As I approached the house to which I had been directed, I found it surrounded by meadows filled with grazing Hereford heifers. 'Hmmm!' I thought. 'This may turn out to be a nice, new account. Real pretty ranch.'

I parked my vehicle and got out. A group of people, including two men in bib overalls, were on the front porch, watching a tethered two-year-old Hereford bull graze on the lawn.

'Howdy, Doc. Pleased to meet you. This here's my brother-in-law, Talbot Heffernan, and there's my wife, Lucille, and Talbot's wife, my sister Anne, and the kids are mine, William and Marylou.'

'Glad to know you,' I said, 'and this must be the bull. He certainly looks normal.'

'Told you so, Doc. Happy as a clam.'

'Are you *sure* he swallowed the hose?'

'Four foot, Doc. Show 'im the bit-off chunk, Talbot.'

Talbot proudly displayed a three-foot-long piece of garden hose, one end bitten through by the bull's sharp molars.

'Well,' I said, 'there's nothing to do but operate – open up his stomach.'

'Well, let's do 'er, then,' said Bob Nesbitt, while Talbot happily nodded his head in agreement.

'I don't see a chute,' I said, looking around. 'We do this operation standing. Do you have a chute?'

'Nope,' said Talbot.

'Well, how do you work the cattle?' I asked.

'What cattle?'

'The cattle,' I said, waving in several directions at the grazing heifers.

'Oh, those aren't *our* cattle,' the Nesbitts chorused.

'They're not?'

'Oh, no! We just got an acre here.'

'But I thought this was a herd sire. I thought you said he was valuable bull.'

'He is, to us,' said Mr Nesbitt. 'He's the only one we own.'

'Well, what are you going to do with him?' I asked, puzzled.

'We gonna *eat* him!' said Talbot. Marylou said, 'Yum, yum! Ah *like* meat!'

'You're going to *eat* him? When?' I asked.

'Oh, in 'bout six months, when he's fattened up.'

'But, if you're raising him for slaughter,' I asked, 'why wasn't he castrated? Why is he still a bull?'

'Nobody told us to,' said Talbot.

'If you're going to butcher him, you want a *steer*, not a bull,' I explained. 'He should have been castrated.'

'Tell you what, Doc,' said Nesbitt. 'Long as you're gonna operate, how 'bout castratin' him at the same time?'

'Wait a minute,' I said. 'When were you planning to slaughter?'

'In October,' said Talbot. 'We're gonna eat 'im in October.'

'Yum,' said Marylou.

'I'll tell you what,' I said. 'I have an idea that will save you a lot of money, and the bull a lot of post-surgical discomfort.'

'What's that?' said the men, together.

'Why don't you eat him *now*?'

'Well, all right,' said Talbot, happily.

'Yum,' said Marylou.

'Thank *you*, Doc, for all you've done. We 'preciate it!'

*　　　*　　　*

Actually it is not all that uncommon for a veterinarian to find himself in a situation not exactly what it originally seemed to be. Usually it all starts with a phone call.

'This is Mr Pearson,' the voice on the telephone said, 'I live on Moorpark Road, and I have a mule I'd like you to geld.'

Arriving at the neat little farmhouse, I was greeted by Mr and Mrs Pearson, an elderly, white-haired couple. The mule was haltered and tied to an oak tree.

'He's two years old and going over fences after my mares,' Mr Pearson explained. 'He really should have been castrated a long time ago.'

I didn't comment, because it is common for people to postpone gelding until long after an animal is mature. I consider this a foolish thing to do because nothing useful is gained by delaying the operation. Horse owners often ask, 'Shouldn't you wait until the animal develops?' I answer, 'Develops what, bad habits?' Nobody can look at a mature gelding and tell whether it was castrated at one week, one month, or one year of age. In my opinion, gelding should be done early, before behavioural problems are established. I gelded my mule when it was three weeks of age.

Working on the lawn, I soon had Mr Pearson's mule anaesthetized and castrated. After cleaning my instruments, I gave Mr Pearson written instructions for post-operative care of the mule. Most important was the recommendation to exercise the mule twice daily for a week, in order to combat swelling and promote drainage from the incision.

Mr and Mrs Pearson, heads close together, read the note and then, in subdued but intense voices, debated my instructions.

'Is there a problem?' I asked. 'You don't have to ride the mule to exercise it. You can lead the mule or work it on a long line or whatever.'

'That's not the problem, Doctor,' explained Mrs Pearson. 'You see, that isn't our mule, it belongs to our neighbour. If we exercise that critter twice a day, the owner might catch us at it and find out what we had done.'

'You mean that this isn't your mule?' I gasped. 'This is your neighbour's mule, and he doesn't know that you planned to have it gelded?'

'That mule has been a pain in the neck,' Mrs Pearson asserted, while her husband nodded his head vigorously. 'It comes over the fences after our mares!'

Mr Pearson added, 'The man who owns the mule is so dumb he'll never notice that it was gelded – unless, of course, he sees us over there exercising his mule.'

'Listen!' I pleaded. 'You didn't tell me this! I don't know anything about it! You asked me to do the surgery, and I did it. Now I'm leaving, and it's up to you to figure out how to exercise the mule.'

I didn't hear any more about the incident, so I assume the owner of the mule never learned that his animal was castrated. On the other hand, perhaps he contrived the entire situation, so his neighbours would pay for the operation.

Chapter 14

At some point in his career, almost every veterinarian will have to work on a wild animal or two. My practice included not only exotic captive species, but native wild animals. Dealing with them often resulted in the unexpected turns that make the work of a veterinarian such a challenge and such an adventure. It is now illegal in California for a veterinarian to de-scent a skunk. This law was passed to reduce the exposure of people to rabid skunks, because this species is our most serious reservoir of rabies virus. Consequently, we no longer see pet skunks, but years ago they were common.

I always felt obligated to de-scent skunks surgically when asked to do so, but frankly, I disliked the task. No matter how careful I was, some odour always permeated my person, the instruments, and the operating room. Horses would shy away from me for a couple of days, and one night when I arrived home long after dark, my own dogs nearly attacked me. Finally I decided to do the surgery out of doors, on an empty lot next to the clinic.

I had two rules about de-scenting skunks: first, I would only operate on immature animals. Older skunks just do not make acceptable pets. They rarely become gentle enough to be handled. Second, I insisted that the client reach into the cage or box and grab the skunk by the tail and lift it into the air. Everyone knew that a skunk cannot squirt when it is hanging by its tail. At least, that is what everybody said.

One day, Marguerite Cummings telephoned. Marguerite was the nineteen-year-old daughter of the owners of a local guest ranch. Tall, voluptuously constructed, blonde, and glamorous. Marguerite favoured form-fitting, expensive clothing. It was fortunate that she lived in the country. In the city she would have been a menace, traipsing about causing automobiles to rear-end other automobiles, and scores of young men to brain themselves by walking into lamp posts. Marguerite was one of those girls who are even more impressive walking away than walking toward one.

'My friend, Peggy, who is a registered nurse – in training – and I have captured a cute little skunk here at the ranch. Will you tell Peggy how to de-scent the skunk?' asked Marguerite.

'Certainly,' I agreed readily, motivated by a combination of amusement and devilment. 'Put your friend on the other phone.'

I then proceeded to describe the procedure. 'Let Marguerite grab the skunk by the tail and hoist it into the air. Then, Peggy, you inject pentobarbital sodium intraperitoneally – one-fourth c.c. per pound of body weight – into the skunk's abdomen. After the skunk is sound asleep, grasp the papillae, which lie somewhat ventrally on either side of the anus, with a curved mosquito haemostatic forceps. With gentle traction, dissect the gland from the skin and surrounding tissues, using a dull Bard-Parker number ten blade. Be very careful not to perforate the wall of the sac. . .'

I described the rest of the surgery, whereupon Peggy suggested to Marguerite, as I anticipated, that 'it sounds complicated. Maybe we ought to let the doctor do it.'

Marguerite reluctantly asked for an appointment.

'How old is the skunk?' I asked.

'We don't know, but he's so cute. He's a real baby!'

'Can you pick him up by the tail so I can inject the anaesthetic?' I asked.

'Oh, certainly. He's easy to handle!'

The next morning Marguerite showed up in a station wagon with a hinged wooden box in the back. She was clad in toreador pants of gold lamé, only two sizes too small. She wore a translucent blouse, a lot of turquoise jewellery. The frames of her harlequin sun glasses were studded with rhinestones. Her long palamino mane gleamed in the sun. Got the picture?

I emerged from my office carrying an instrument tray and anaesthetic equipment. 'We'll work on the tailgate of your wagon,' I said as I loaded my syringe. 'Will you please lift him out of the box by his tail?'

'Me?' asked Marguerite.

'Yes. I told you that you would have to do that so I could inject the anaesthetic. You did say you had handled him before, didn't you?'

'Oh, sure,' Marguerite answered, somewhat dubiously. Then she opened the lid of the box and peered in. 'Hi, Flower!' she said. 'Nice boy!' She quickly reached in and pulled out the biggest old boar skunk I had ever seen. Rolling off the tailgate of the wagon, she jumped to the ground and faced me, shrieking, 'Here! Quick! Do something!'

'Hey!' I protested. 'You said he was a cute little. . .'

The skunk's feet paddled wildly. His beady black eyes gleamed satanically. He was as large as a house cat, fat and black and white. Marguerite leaned forward, right arm in the air dangling the skunk, left arm stretched behind her, fingers outspread spastically.

The skunk revolved clockwise as far as its tail permitted and then began revolving slowly in the opposite direction. As it did so, the skunk squirted a yellow fog right across Marguerite's translucent blouse.

I was interested to note two things. First, that the air was immediately filled with a stunning, overwhelming odour. I remember thinking what a marvellous protective device this was, and that although I had smelled skunk scent many times, I had never fully appreciated its efficacy when emitted as a fine aerosol under high pressure. I was downwind, and I will always be proud of the lightning-fast reflexes that propelled me in a single bound out of the prevailing breeze, toward the front of the car. Second, despite the urgency of the situation, I could not help noticing that Marguerite's blouse, when wet, was not translucent. It was transparent.

'Ugh!' screamed Marguerite. 'Oh! Oh! Oh!' She lifted the skunk higher into the air. Everybody knows that skunks can only squirt once, but Marguerite was not taking any chances. If the skunk fired again, she did not want another charge on her Maidenform.

The skunk, having completed its clockwise revolution, began to revolve back in its original direction. As it approached the one-hundred-and-eighty-degree (or six-o'clock) position, it fired both barrels! Marguerite caught the charge directly in the face – right across the lenses of the harlequin sun glasses. In response, she said something that sounded like 'Ugh! Ugh! Ugh! Ugh!'

With marvellous discipline (she never dropped the skunk) Marguerite climbed back into the wagon, gasping, retching, dripping, and stinking, to deposit Flower in the crate.

'So!' I thought. 'Skunks can express their scent glands when held by the tail, and they can do it more than once!'

My scientific reverie was broken by the sight of Marguerite standing before me, making inarticulate sounds, hunched over, half-blinded by the spattered sun glasses, hands outspread.

Filled with compassion – or perhaps it was guilt – I made the mistake of suggesting she come into the clinic to clean up. Leading the poor blinded girl at arm's length, I took her inside. For more than a week I regretted that move. The odour permeated the entire building. Only time eventually removed it.

Finally I was relieved to steer the girl back to her station wagon. 'Go home,' I suggested. 'Turn the skunk loose. Burn your clothes, and take a bath in tomato juice. Wash your hair in it!'

'Tomato juice?' she whined.

'Yes,' I assured her. 'It's the best thing to neutralize the odour. That's what we do for dogs that have tangled with a skunk. We dip them in tomato juice.'

The sight of Cleopatra in a bath of milk inspired Mark Antony. I still laugh as I picture Marguerite soaking in a tub of tomato juice.

It was late on Christmas Eve when Jack Chambers, a professional writer, phoned. 'Doc,' he said, 'I hate to bother you at such a time, but I just came across a wounded fox. It's still alive, but unconscious. Can I bring it in?'

I met Jack at the clinic and examined a comatose California grey fox showing signs of intra-cranial haemorrhage. A wheel must have gone over its head.

'I'll pay the charges,' Jack said. 'Do what you can for it.'

'This is a wild animal,' I reminded him. 'If it starts to recover, handling it will be dangerous.'

'Please,' said Jack, 'I feel so sorry for it. Do what you can to try to save it.'

Apprehensively, I began therapy. For two days, the fox was kept in intensive care and fed intravenously. Then, gradually, it started lifting its head. Soon it could swallow when spoon fed. It made no attempt to bite.

On the fourth day, I told Mr and Mrs Chambers I felt they could care for the fox at home. But I warned them that once the fox was sufficiently recovered, it would probably start biting because of fear. Filled with Christmas spirit, my partner and I split the bill with the Chamberses.

During the next few weeks, the fox, now named 'Daryl the Twentieth Century Fox,' made a remarkable recovery. At the end of two weeks, Daryl seemed to be normal except for three deficiencies. First, he apparently had lost his sense of smell. When food was placed in his mouth he ate greedily, but he seemed unaware of its presence even if the dish was put right in front of him.

Second, Daryl was blind. His eyes looked normal, except for a squint in the left one, but his brain could not interpret what his eyes perceived, and he was oblivious to all visual stimuli.

Last, Daryl had lost all aggressiveness and hostility. He cringed in fear when touched, but never attempted to bite.

'It's as though he's had a lobotomy,' said Jack. 'He's incapable of attacking.'

A veterinary neurologist we consulted agreed. 'The geniculate ganglion and adjacent areas were apparently severely damaged in the accident,' he theorized. 'He may recover some day, and if and when he does, he will probably revert to his wild ferocity.'

One day, Daryl was brought to the office to see us. Although timid, he was now a tame house pet. He loved to ride in the car, ate without help, was house-broken, walked on a leash, and enjoyed being groomed. He had lost his wild odour, and he played with the family cat.

We went outdoors so I could take pictures of Daryl. When a client drove up and got out of her car with a large dog, Daryl turned toward the dog and crouched, his pupils dilated widely. Daryl could see! His vision had returned, and from that day on, he was a normal fox except for his total lack of aggressiveness.

The Chamberses took Daryl on a cross-country trip. He had become a beloved but mischievous pet. His favourite prank was to race about the house, overturning the waste baskets.

One day in June, half a year after the accident, a friend of the Chamberses came to visit. She approached Daryl, who was curled up on the mantel over the fireplace. 'Daryl!' she addressed him. 'How is my little friend?' She reached out to stroke the fox. Without warning, he whipped his head toward her hand and bit her finger. From that moment on Daryl attempted to bite anyone who touched him. A few days later, he disappeared.

Daryl had been gone two weeks when he was seen again. Jack was driving home one evening and saw a fox in a meadow near the road. The fox was wearing the collar the Chamberses had bought for Daryl. Jack got out of the car and called, 'Daryl, come boy! Come!' The fox looked at Jack for half a minute, then ran into the brush.

The Chamberses never saw their fox again, but they came home one evening and found all the waste baskets overturned. Apparently Daryl had entered through an open window, explored his former home, and returned to the wild. His former friend, the cat, was in the house, unscathed.

About a year later, I was on a call to a little ranch high up in Decker canyon, the place where Daryl had been run over.

I treated an Angus heifer. Then the owner asked me, 'Doctor, what does a rabid fox act like? We've got a fox around here that comes up to the house, gets up on the window sill, and looks in through the glass. But just as soon as we step outside, he runs of as fast as he can. This has happened four or five times.'

'Did he have a collar on?' I asked.

90

'No, why would he be wearing a collar?'

I told him the story of Daryl the Twentieth Century Fox, and we agreed that the fox he was seeing must be Daryl. How confused that animal must have been, torn between his wild instincts and the fading memory of human kindness.

Chapter 15

Millions of Americans have dogs as pets, usually for the simple reason that they bring so much joy to their owners.

During the early days of television a basset hound named Cleo popularized that formerly exotic breed. One of my clients at that time was a recently widowed woman. Both she and her deceased husband were the kind of people who make practice a joy. They were always pleasant, appreciative, considerate, and smiling. And they paid their bills conscientiously, although they were obviously not affluent. The widow had not been left in a financially secure position when her husband died. In fact, in order to make ends meet and to allow her teen-aged daughter to complete high school, the woman had taken a job as a waitress.

The mother and daughter were strongly attached to their ailing pet cat, so I saw them often. One day the woman said, 'Dr Miller, we are lonesome at home with Dad gone, and Tommy is old and sick half the time as you know, so we've been thinking about getting a dog. You must run across situations where people have to give up a dog, or perhaps an injured stray is brought in.'

I assured them that we frequently had dogs in the hospital that needed a home for one reason or another.

'Will you let us know when you find one suitable for us? We're not in a hurry, and we'll leave the selection entirely up to you.'

I readily agreed to find them a dog, and then asked what kind of dog they'd like.

They looked at each other and smiled with some embarrassment. The daughter explained, 'Well, we don't really expect to get the kind of dog we'd really like to have, because we priced a few pups and that kind of dog is just too expensive for us. We decided to settle for any kind of medium-sized dog, with not too shaggy a coat, because we live in an apartment. We considered adopting one from the pound, but you know us, and we'd have more confidence if you found one for us. We've never had a dog before – just cats.'

'But what kind of dog was it you shopped for? What breed?' I asked the daughter, a polite, pretty sixteen-year-old. The mother answered, 'She's just crazy about Cleo. You know, the basset hound on TV? We both are! We'd give anything to own a dog like that, but of course, we don't expect you to find anything so valuable for us. A nice mongrel will do.'

The daughter suggested, 'I wouldn't mind a dog with floppy ears and sad eyes, but anything you pick out for us will be fine.'

I promised to remember and to place the first appropriate homeless pup with them.

A few weeks later, a basset breeder came in with a four-month-old female. 'I want her put to sleep. Her front feet splay out badly, and I have to cull her,' the breeder explained.

I suggested that we place the pup, *sans* registration papers, as a pet. 'I even have a home in mind,' I offered. Then I told the breeder about the widow and daughter.

She agreed to give me the pup, but first made me swear that I would not reveal where it came from or what its blood line was.

After examining the puppy, immunizing it, and finding it to be sweet and gentle, I phoned the widow at work.

'I have a dog for you,' I told her. She was delighted and promised to come in before our office closed.

At 5:30 p.m. the lady and her daughter showed up, eyes sparkling with excitement.

'I have a dog for you – a female – and I think you'll be pleased,' I said with careful indifference. I was savouring the surprise I had for these nice people.

'What kind of dog is she?' asked the woman.

'How old is she?' asked the daughter.

'I've examined her and she's fine, and she's had all her vaccinations,' I responded.

'How old is she?' asked the widow.

'How big is she?' asked the daughter.

'If you're not happy with her, you're free to return her,' I said, 'but I'm confident that you'll become very fond of her.'

'Where is she?' asked the widow.

'Can we see her?' asked the daughter.

I continued, 'The present owner cannot keep her, and so, if you like her, she is yours to keep, forever.'

The daughter wrung her hands. 'Can we see her, Doctor Miller? Where is she?'

'Oh,' I suddenly recalled. 'Before we go on about this dog, I have something else for you. One of the drug companies sent me a series of dog portraits, and one of them is of a basset puppy. I remember that you told me you wished you could have one. Since that isn't possible, I thought you'd like to have this picture.'

All thoughts of the dog in the back room were put aside as they viewed the photograph of the irresistible little hound.

'Oh, Mom! Look at that! Oh, isn't that the most adorable thing you've ever seen in your life!'

Soon the mother interjected, 'Honey, the doctor is busy. We'd better see what kind of a real dog he's found for us and take it on home.'

I led them into the kennel room, and still keeping them in suspense and ignoring the barrage of questions they fired at me, I reached deliberately into a cage. Turning around I deposited the enormous-eared, loose-skinned, tricoloured puppy in the daughter's arms.

I wasn't prepared for their reaction. Happy smiles gave way to tears. Mother and daughter hugged each other, the puppy, and the picture I had given them, and cried. I heard and saw simultaneous joy and sorrow, both expressed in tears. Soon I too had tears streaming down my face.

The puppy, in gratitude, was named Roberta and, of course, lived happily ever after.

Of all my canine patients, I'd say my favourite was Pal. He belonged to Gerald Davis, a local working cowboy. Pal was a nondescript Australian shepherd possessed of one 'glass' (blue) eye, a short, bristly, muddy merle coat, the ability to climb trees, and the brains of a twelve-year-old human.

Pal worked cattle on the rugged and sprawling Conejo Ranch. In the spring and early summer, the California grasses are decorated with seeds, all of which are equipped with barbed penetrating awns and are grouped under common nomenclature as 'foxtails.' The foxtails have a special affinity for the ear canals of dogs. During foxtail season, Gerald would bring Pal to the office on Monday morning to have the preceding week's collection of foxtail bristles removed from his ears, a painful procedure.

'Get up on the table,' Gerald would suggest, and the good dog promptly complied. 'Hold still while the doctor takes out the foxtails.'

Pal would squint and wince, but unheld by human hands, would never move until I had removed a dozen or so bristly seeds from each ear. Then I'd say, 'That does it,' whereupon Pal would reach around, lick my hand once in a gesture of gratitude and then calmly jump off the table.

'Go wait for me in the truck,' Gerald would suggest. Pal would then, by himself, walk laconically to the front door and, when let out, proceed to the battered pickup and jump in.

Sadly, this marvellous dog tangled with a less friendly truck and was killed on the highway. A great dog was lost.

Bruno was a handsome three-year-old male boxer with an exceptional disposition and a stoic temperament. But Charles and Janet Webster looked worried.

'We just moved out here from the city,' Mr Webster, a young man of about thirty, told me. 'Our old veterinarian has been treating Bruno for kennel cough, but he doesn't seem to be getting any better. In fact, he's worse. This is the third week he's had this low fever and a cough, and he's losing weight. He's been on several different antibiotics and cough medicine, but they don't seem to help.'

I telephoned Doctor Davidson, the veterinarian who had been caring for the dog.

'It looked like plain old tracheobronchitis,' he explained. 'I used the usual kennel-cough treatment, but if he's still sick after all this time, I don't know. I saw him three times. Maybe I'm missing something. He is a boxer, and they are highly susceptible to malignancy. Maybe I've missed a chest tumour. You'd better take some chest X-rays.'

I examined Bruno. He was bright enough and wagged his stump of a tail as I went over him, but there was something ominous about his retching cough and the way his ribs showed because of recent weight loss. His temperature was slightly elevated.

'One-oh-three,' I said, reading the thermometer. 'He hasn't been in the desert recently, has he?' I asked.

The Websters looked up quickly. 'Why, yes! We were in Phoenix a few weeks ago. Bruno had a grand time exploring the desert, chasing lizards and gophers and all. How did you know?'

'There's a fungal infection in southwestern deserts,' I explained, 'and boxer dogs are especially susceptible to it. It's called coccidioidal mycosis, or Valley Fever. I'd like to take some chest X-rays and run some tests on Bruno.'

Bruno did indeed have coccidioidal mycosis. I had made a clever diagnosis, but I was not pleased. First of all, it is easy to be a superior diagnostician after some other veterinarian has done the preliminary work. When Bruno failed to respond to conventional treatment, it was obvious that he was suffering from an unconventional disease. Secondly, I had practised in southern Arizona before coming to California. I had seen quite a few cases of Valley Fever. Lastly, I knew Bruno was going to die and that losing him was going to break his owners' hearts. Few dogs survive a full-blown case of pulmonary coccidioidal mycosis, and all of the boxers I had seen with the disease had died.

'Can't anything be done?' Mr Webster asked grimly. His wife wept silently. I had just shown them the radiographs and told them that the tests were positive.

'There is a drug used to treat this disease. It's called amphotericin B,' I said. 'But, unfortunately, it is a very toxic drug, and it usually damages the kidneys so severely that the patients die of uremia before they die of the fungus.'

'Let's try it anyway,' said Mr Webster. Mrs Webster nodded in agreement as he added, 'Bruno is a very special dog, and he means a great deal to us. We want to give him any chance there is, however remote.'

Bruno was hospitalized and the staff soon understood why his owners loved him dearly. No better patient could be imagined. The drug was administered intravenously, by means of a slow drip. Bruno was put on a treatment table, hooked up to the intravenous drip and told to stay. There he would stay. For two long hours that gentlemanly dog stayed on the table, never attempting to jump off without permission, never removing the needle or tubing from his leg. He sat there, silent, dignified, wagging his tail slowly when approached. A special dog indeed.

For a while, Bruno's condition seemed to improve. With every treatment we ran a blood urea nitrogen test. Soon, the values began to rise. Bruno's kidneys were being destroyed by the drug, even before the drug destroyed the fungus in his system.

As time went on and as Bruno's kidneys increasingly deteriorated, his appetite disappeared. He grew emaciated and nauseated.

'We can't go on with the drug,' I told the Websters. 'The fungus is still active in his body, but the treatment has now damaged his kidneys, possibly beyond repair. We are so very sorry. He is a wonderful dog – a noble dog. But we cannot do any more for him.'

Mr Webster hesitated. 'Is he suffering?' he asked.

'He's not in pain, I answered, 'but he feels very, very sick. He is weak and nauseated, and his lung infection makes it difficult for him to breathe. If Bruno were mine, I'd do the humane thing, but you must make that decision yourself.'

Charles Webster pondered silently. He had left his wife at home. 'I just can't do it yet,' he said with a broken voice. 'I'll take him home and make his remaining time as comfortable as possible. When he looks beyond hope, or if we feel he is suffering, we'll put him to sleep.'

Bruno went home, wrapped in a blanket. The once powerfully muscled body was now pitifully thin. His chest heaved with each breath. As he panted, his pale blue tongue hung from his mouth. His eyes were sunken and listless. Bruno was dying.

Several days went by. I thought of Bruno several times, meaning to phone the Websters, but always became immersed in a myriad of other cases.

Then Charles Webster called me. 'Doctor Miller,' he said, 'Bruno is near death, and we feel that it is time to put him to sleep. He just lies there almost in a coma and has to be helped to his feet. He has lost control over his bowels and bladder.'

I told Mr Webster that I felt he was doing the right thing. 'Bring him down,' I advised.

'Well, we want to do something first. You see, Bruno is such a fantastic dog, we always wanted a pup sired by him.

97

We planned to breed him when he grew old, and keep a pup so we'd have a replacement for him, but we never expected to lose him this early. There's a boxer bitch down the street in season right now. Her owner is willing to let Bruno breed her, but he wants you to call him and reassure him that there is no danger of his female catching Valley Fever from Bruno.'

'I'll do that,' I responded, 'but Bruno sounds terminal. What makes you think he'd have either the strength or the desire to mate?'

'Doctor,' said Mr Webster, 'Bruno is a gentleman, but a very masculine gentleman. We may have to hold him up, but if I know my dog, he'll breed that female.'

When I came into the office the following week, there was a note on my desk to call Mr Webster.

'Bruno died during the night,' he said.

'I'm sorry,' I answered. 'I know it has been an ordeal for you, and I regret that you didn't get one of his pups before he got sick.'

'Oh, he said, 'But we'll get our pup. Bruno bred that bitch a few days before he died.'

Four months later the Websters came to the clinic. In Mrs Webster's arms was a sturdy two-month-old male boxer puppy. I took him and put him on the examination table. Most boxer pups are wriggly and effusively friendly. This one eyed me calmly. Dignity and patience marked his wrinkled little face. The stub tail wagged a quiet greeting.

'We call him Bruno,' said Janet Webster.

Although my diagnosis of Bruno had been quick and on the mark, I also had, as all veterinarians do, my share of difficult cases.

When I had the time for such things, I enjoyed doing clinical trials for various pharmaceutical companies. Many of the products I tested were disappointing. Others were effective, but were never marketed. The majority, however, were subsequently introduced to the profession, and many are now staples in the veterinarian armamentarium. One such product is Squibb's Panalog®, an ear and topical ointment known to every practitioner.

The supply of Panalog I received was labelled as an experimental product and identified by a code number. I don't believe the trade name had been selected at this stage.

Mrs Regal was a wealthy and aristocratic lady who owned a thoroughbred horse ranch in Hidden Valley, a lush and pastoral valley just south of Thousand Oaks. Mrs Regal also owned an Irish setter. The dog was aging and had formed the familiar habit of constantly licking one of its forepaws until a nasty-looking lesion called a lick granuloma developed. I was anxious to make a favourable impression on Mrs Regal, in the hope that she would consider my services for her fine horses.

'I have an excellent new product which, I think, will help heal that lesion,' I said. I dispensed several tubes of the Squibb ointment with instructions to apply it daily and keep the lesion covered with a protective bandage.

Two weeks later, I saw Mrs Regal again in my office. 'That yellow ointment accomplished nothing,' she said. 'Sport's sore looks worse than before. What else do you suggest?'

I examined the lesion again, uncomfortably. It was really too large to excise surgically. 'I've had some success treating these with intradermal injections of cortisone,' I said. 'Let's try that next.'

'Whatever you think will work best, Doctor,' said the lady. 'Sport is a dear old friend, and we'll do anything to make him well.'

Accordingly, I treated the setter's paw in this manner and asked to see him again in two weeks. Mrs Regal kept the appointment, but to my great discomfort, the granuloma was unchanged.

'What do we do now?' asked the owner in a somewhat critical tone.

'I'd like to try some X-ray therapy,' I offered. 'Some of these lesions respond dramatically to radiation.'

'Do whatever you think will help Sport,' said Mrs Regal.

My diagnostic X-ray machine had been calibrated by a radiation physicist for superficial therapy. I treated the paw three times. Each treatment required general anaesthesia.

The paw looked exactly the same after the treatment had been completed.

'I think my equipment is inadequate for a lesion as deep as this one looks,' I explained. 'Would you mind driving to Santa Monica? I want to refer you to a colleague who has an X-ray therapy machine. I'm sure he could get better results.'

'I'd drive to New York if it would help Sport,' said Mrs Regal.

Sport underwent a series of X-ray therapy treatments in Santa Monica. Each treatment was performed under anaesthesia. The paw looked the same.

Mrs Regal was haughtily patient. 'What else can we try?' she asked.

We tried an evil-tasting cream to discourage Sport from licking. Then we put a basket muzzle on him. He managed to lick through the muzzle. We tried tranquillizers. He licked more slowly, but continued to lick. We tried proprietary healing ointments. We took a biopsy of the lesion; it was a lick granuloma. It would not heal. Sport was fitted with a leather boot which covered the lesion. He licked a hole in the leather, exposing the sore underneath. We tried exercise and invented games to relieve his boredom. I suggested he follow Mrs Regal when she rode horseback through the hills. Sport came back from the rides with his tongue lolling out, flopped down, and commenced licking his paw. I telephoned colleagues for advice. We tried tonics, supplements, and corrective compounds. Sport licked with greater energy. I consulted dermatology tests. I wrote a prescription for an exotic coal tar formula. Sport licked them all. I began to suspect that the soulful-looking dog was involved in a diabolical plot to embarrass me in the eyes of his wealthy owner. Mrs Regal, amazingly, never seemed to despair of my futile efforts. She came in with Sport regularly, paid her bills, and patiently tried each idea I came up with.

Finally, I suggested that the lesion be surgically excised and the resulting skin defect be repaired with a graft.

Mrs Regal wanted to think about this. She took Sport home and never brought him back. For nearly a year, she had admirably maintained her confidence in my inadequate efforts. Now, at last, she had abandoned me. How could I blame her? I blushed every time I drove by the gate to her ranch.

Many months passed. Then, one day, as I approached the post office, I met Mrs Regal coming out of the doorway. 'Good morning,' I greeted her. 'Say, Mrs Regal, how is old Sport doing?'

'Oh, he's quite well for an old man,' she replied sweetly.

'Uh, how is that paw?' I asked.

'It's completely healed,' she offered enthusiastically. 'As good as new!'

'Really?' I asked in surprise. 'What finally did the trick?'

Mrs Regal looked at me for a moment, her face a study in speculation and pity.

'I finally took Sport to Doctor Parizo in Oxnard,' she said. Ernie Parizo was a classmate of mine about twenty miles down the road.

'Panolog!' exclaimed Mrs Regal. 'It's a new product. Just came on the market. Spelled P-A-N-O-L-O-G. Try it, young man. I think you'll find it useful.'

Chapter 16

Bud Spavin is a farrier. My practice was only a few months old when I met him. I had been called to see a horse with an eye problem. When I arrived, Bud was shoeing another horse nearby.

The owner led my patient out of the barn. One eye was swollen and runny. The cornea was cloudy and inflamed. After identifying an ulcer with fluorescein stain, I said, 'We should have begun treating this eye a week ago, when the injury happened.'

The owner explained, 'I did treat it. I put KIP® in the eye every day!'

'What is KIP?' I asked. She produced a tube of ointment. 'Why, this isn't an eye ointment!' I protested after reading the label. 'This is for sunburn!'

The farrier straightened up and glared at me. He spat on the ground, strode towards us, grabbed the tube of KIP and growled, 'Hell, Doc, I've been using this stuff in eyes for years!' He then pulled one of his lower eyelids down with a grimy forefinger and squirted a great gob of the ointment into his own eye. I gaped speechlessly while he glared malevolently at me with his visible eye, the other now obscured by the white cream smeared over his entire cornea.

He spat again and marched away muttering. 'Damn! KIP ain't gonna hurt that eye!'

I did not see Bud for several months. Then one day I made a call to a ranch in the hills. The owner grazed a herd of buffalo and assorted cattle. He had caught a big, horned Holstein cow. She was range-bred and wild as a deer. Planning to sell this animal, the owner needed a brucellosis blood test. The corral was not equipped with a chute.

'How am I going to bleed her without a chute?' I asked the owner.

I didn't realize it, but Bud lived in a house trailer on this ranch. He suddenly appeared from behind a pickup truck. 'Why you'll just have to rope her, Doc,' he sneered. 'You know how to handle cattle don't you?'

Not answering, I got my lariat from my car. The cow's horns stuck up, visible over the fences. She was separated from me by two fences which formed a fifteen-foot lane used for moving cattle. She did not see me throw a back-hand loop. By the greatest of luck it settled right around her horns. I snubbed the cow to a post and looked at the men. The old rancher was grinning, and Bud's mouth and eyes were wide. 'Did you see that? He caught her horns over two fences. That's about as good as a man can do!' The rancher said.

From that moment on, Bud became an admirer. He had decided that I was worthless because I didn't use KIP as an eye ointment. Now he decided that I was a brilliant veterinarian because of a lucky throw with a rope. Bud never let logic interfere with an opinion.

Although aging, Bud is still around, still shoeing horses. Our relationship is amicable, but professionally we are at odds. He regards the horse, from the fetlock down, as his sole province. No matter what type of shoe I prescribe for a horse, Bud, if he is the farrier, will stubbornly ignore my instructions. If I request a high heel, he lowers it, and vice versa. I explain this to the owner, and then reverse my instructions. The horse improves. Bud is happy. The owner is happy. I am happy.

Once Bud called me to see a bunch of his own cattle that had severe ulcerative pinkeye. I suggested he treat them with KIP. 'That don't help pinkeye, Doc!' he bellowed. 'I want some of the stuff you used on Turnbull's cattle!' Having trapped him into accepting my therapy, I prescribed atropine and chloramphenicol ophthalmic ointments.

Bud has one of those independent, self-sufficient frontier personalities that are gradually disappearing from the American scene. He castrated his own colts, roping their front feet, tying them down, and performing the gelding

103

operation without benefit of a pain killer.

Therefore, I was surprised one day when Bud called me to geld a colt, but shortly after I arrived, he defensively explained, 'This ain't my colt, Doc. If it was, I'da cut him myself. The lady who owns him wanted a vet. Suits me! Must like to spend money. Shoot, I cut a million of 'em! Forefoot 'em and bust 'em and cut 'em before they know what hit 'em.'

As I tranquillized the colt and selected my instrument Bud kept up the barrage. 'Can't see makin' a big deal out of a simple operation. Rope 'em, put a good man on the head, cut 'em one-two-three, and run 'em back out. Get on them the next day and ride the hell out of 'em. Does 'em good! Sure don't need a college education to cut colts! No big deal.'

I took succinylcholine chloride out of the truck refrigerator and filled a 2-c.c. syringe. Succinylcholine chloride is a paralysing drug. If given intravenously to a horse, the animal will, in a couple of minutes, start to show twitching called fasciculation. Then the horse will abruptly collapse, completely paralysed. The paralysis lasts for a few minutes, after which the horse regains its feet. For twenty years this drug was widely used by veterinarians doing horse practice. I used succinylcholine most frequently for castrating colts, combining it with a pain-relieving drug.

Seeing me fill the syringe, Bud said, 'Good idea, give him a tetanus shot first! I always give 'em a tetanus shot. Never cut a colt and had it get tetanus. Good idea!'

From somewhere deep in the depths of my depraved mind, an idea glowed. No, it was not an idea; it was an inspiration! And it was growing! I trembled with mischievous glee.

In the cab of my pickup was an ultrasound-therapy machine destined for use on a later patient. I removed it and handed the end of a long extension cord to Bud. 'Mind plugging this in?' I asked.

Bud complied, marching off grumbling. I stepped up to the sedated colt and quickly injected the succinylcholine.

'Good idea, tetanus,' Bud repeated.

Nonchalantly I returned to the truck, discarded the syringe, and picked up the head of the ultrasound machine. About eight seconds had passed since I had given the injection. I switched on the machine, turning it on high, and poured a few drops of surgical soap on the face of the head. Another five seconds had passed. The soap boiled furiously as the ultra-high frequency sound waves hit the liquid. Bud's eyebrows elevated. He watched with silent interest. Suddenly, I turned to face the colt, holding the machine head in both hands like a policeman firing a magnum. Still pointing the machine, I raised up on my toes dramatically, like a matador about to face the moment of truth.

Bud murmured, 'Doc, do you wear a hat out in the sun? You know. . .'

Abruptly the colt's eyelids flashed. His muscles started to twitch, first over the shoulders and then progressively back over his body. Bud stopped talking. In fact, behind me, I heard him stop breathing. The colt dropped spectacularly to the ground.

I switched off the machine and ran to the colt. Quickly, I performed the castration. Bud was silent. The colt regained his feet. I gathered up my equipment, cleaned it up, and put it away. Bud stood by, still speechless, his face a mask of awe and respect. Finally, I unplugged the machine and carried it to the cab. Bud eyed it warily and quickly backed out of my way.

'No rope burns,' I said. Bud was silent but his eyebrows shot up quizzically.

'No rope burns,' I repeated. 'Nice way to put them down.' He looked at me with a mixture of astonishment, deference, and dread.

As I drove away he lifted his hand in a hesitant farewell, still unable to speak. The poor man was overwhelmed.

I knew, at last, what it must feel to be a witch doctor.

Although the lariat has often served me well in a career spent working with animals, it has also been the source of many mishaps.

I learned to throw the rope working on western ranches when I was young. With practice I became reasonably proficient at catching things. Although I rarely won anything, I had a passion for roping and was active in inter-collegiate rodeo.

Until I finished my preveterinary work at the University of Arizona, my roping was confined to horses and cattle. Well, there were a few chickens, goats, and, once a coyote that came within range, but the critters I roped were mostly conventional.

In veterinary school at Colorado, my roping was again conventional. There were summers on Colorado ranches, school rodeos, and occasional targets among patients at the campus hospital.

After I graduated, my repertoire grew. There were, at times, horses and livestock that had to be caught to be treated and a variety of exotic species. In a practice that included circus and zoo animals and 'wild' animal farms, I roped zebra, bison, deer, antelope, leopards, bears, sea lions, ostriches – creatures of almost every conceivable species. I even roped a pilot whale. This has been going on for decades, and continues today.

I may hold some kind of world record for having roped the widest assortment of creatures. When I rope something I have never roped before, I mentally add it to my 'list' like a bird-watcher or a trophy hunter on safari. Roping satisfies the primeval hunting instinct without injuring the quarry. But, as I said, there have been mishaps.

A couple of years after I established my practice in Thousand Oaks, the movie star Lana Turner called me. She had a ranch thirty miles away and wanted a thoroughbred yearling filly treated for an abscess. When I arrived at the ranch, nobody except the actress's mother was at home. The filly was in a half-acre corral, surrounded by a six-foot high chain-link fence.

'Glad you could come, Doctor,' the lady said. 'This is a ten-thousand-dollar filly, and we're worried about her swollen jaw.'

'Okay,' I answered. 'Can you catch her for me?'

'Not on your life,' she retorted. 'I'm not going in there!'

'Oh?' I said, surprised. 'Well, I'll see if I can catch her.'

I not only could not catch the filly; I could not get within twenty feet of her. I had come so far that I hated to leave without treating the animal. When carrots and grain failed as bait, I went to my station wagon for my rope.

'I'll catch her,' I assured the worried woman.

Catch her I did, with a long throw that filled me with pride. The filly was running when I caught her, and I lost the end of the rope. She stampeded around the corral, dragging the lariat.

'She'll slow down soon, and I'll have her,' I explained confidently.

The end of the rope flailed behind the filly. Somehow it snared the guy wire at the top of the fence. instantly the wire tore loose. Now the filly had thirty feet of rope plus fifty feet of singing wire chasing her. Her speed accelerated to a wild sprint. The wire crossed my path, and I jumped into the air to avoid it. After two panic-stricken laps around the corral, the filly made straight for the fence, attempted to jump it, hung briefly from the top of it, then tumbled over it.

Hysterical visions of disembowelment, broken necks, and malpractice suits crossed my mind. Miraculously, the filly rose and stood quietly in shocked silence outside the corral. I caught her and found a couple of minor scratches on her belly. After treating these and the abscessed jaw, I returned the filly to the corral. Then I set to work repairing the fence.

Years later, when I was older and should have been much wiser, I went to a quarter-horse ranch owned by entertainer Buddy Ebsen to vaccinate the foal crop. When I arrived, the owner's daughter said, 'They're all gentle and halter-broken, Doctor, except for that bay filly over there. She's wild as a deer. I've never been able to catch her.'

'Don't worry,' I reassured her. 'We'll catch her!'

Out came my rope. The filly ran along the fence of the half-acre corral, and after two unsuccessful attempts, I dropped a loop around the animal's neck. She was running at top speed, and as the rope caught her, she veered toward me. I waved at her, expecting her to avoid me. Instead she slammed into me.

I had often wondered what it must feel like to be hit by a 300-pound football lineman with a full force. I found out. I got up to find that the anterior cruciate and medial collateral ligaments of my left knee had been ruptured. That loop cost me an operation, a week in the hospital, two months in a hip-length cast, three months away from large-animal practice, nearly an entire ski season, and five thousand dollars.

By the following spring I was ambulatory again. I went to a circus training lot to treat a zebra. The zebra was in a pen with a yak, which resembled a small bison with the horns of a Texas longhorn steer. The zebra was gentle, as zebras go, but the yak was crazy wild.

After treating the zebra, I removed its halter. 'Oh,' the trainer said. 'You should have left it on! I'll never be able to catch her again.'

'I'm sorry,' I apologized, 'I'll catch her and put the halter back on.'

Out came my trusty rope, unused for so many months. It felt good in my hand. I caught the zebra and replaced the halter. As I walked toward the gate, the yak thundered past me. I had just recoiled my rope, and I could not resist the temptation: I flipped the rope out and caught both of the yak's hind legs. He quickly kicked loose, and as I approached the gate I grinned at the trainer and circus hands outside the pen. 'Well, now I can say that I roped a yak!'

Their smiles turned to wide-eyed horror. Behind me I heard thundering hooves. I did not look back. I knew what was there. I jumped for the fence and vaulted over it, barely escaping the enraged yak!

108

'You know, Doctor,' the trainer said, 'if that woolly devil got you down, he'd knee you and hook you like a buffalo.'

I did a lot of thinking the next few minutes, and then I made a vow. Never again, as long as I practise, would I ever use that damned rope to catch another animal – unless, of course, it could not be caught by conventional means.

Chapter 17

We hear stories about people who die because they had no will to live and, conversely, about individuals who overcame impossible physical odds because of an extraordinary will to live. Well, animals are the same way. The will to live varies greatly among animal patients. Some of this variation is breed or species related. For example, I find Arabian horses extremely tenacious of life. On the other hand, collie dogs often fold up when sick or injured and become depressed. I think that the less tenacious patients are better off at home when seriously afflicted, rather than left in a hospital. Some cats have an astounding will to live, whereas sheep often just give up and die. Llamas, in my experience, while tough when it comes to surviving environmental stresses, usually don't fight back when struck down by illness.

Once, I attended a German shepherd that had been hit by a car. Its back had been broken and its spinal cord severed. The poor dog was paraplegic, and the owners refused to accept what had happened. They pleaded for us to 'try.' We explained the permanency and the hopelessness of the injury, but they kept the dog in the hospital where we fed it, and nursed it, and cleaned up after it. After a couple of weeks, the shepherd's hindquarters were quite atrophied, but the owners could not bring themselves to put him to sleep. 'He is so alert, and his front end seems so normal,' they rationalized. Yet, they would not take him home. Somehow, they hoped, a miracle would occur, and they would come to the hospital to see their friend, and the doctor would say, 'I have good news for you. Teddy's paralysis is improving, and we think he will be able to walk again.'

I found it difficult to stay in the ward when the family came to visit the dog. He whined softly to them, his eager licking and his intelligent brown eyes telling of his distress at being separated from them, of his loneliness and pain.

When Teddy's cage was cleaned, he was transferred to a pen. He would pathetically drag his paralysed body around the pen, using his strong forelegs.

One day, while Teddy was in the pen, I saw a sight which startled me and choked me with emotion. Teddy was standing on his forelimbs. His paralysed, withered hind end dangled uselessly, and he balanced, standing, on his forelegs. By the next day, Teddy was walking. He balanced on his forelimbs and *walked* around the pen.

The brave dog's family came to see him. They silently watched their pet lift himself and walk to them, his paralysed rear half swinging from side to side.

'That's disgusting,' said the man.

'Horrible!' said the wife. 'Let's put him to sleep. I can't stand to watch that.'

In a quarter century of veterinary practice, the most courageous animal I have ever known is an Arabian stallion I shall call 'Sheik.'

Sheik foundered back East, so badly that his hooves sloughed away. The bones of his feet rotated and began to disintegrate. Veterinary surgeons rebuilt his feet with acrylic plastics. Deep infections developed, and pus oozed from his soles and from the coronet, where the hair meets the hoof.

The horse's pain was so extreme that, despite prodigious doses of pain-killing drugs, he spent most of his time lying down in the box stall. He arose only with the greatest effort, his feet stuck out in front of him in a salaam that was a grotesque caricature of his Arabian ancestry.

The horse was, after a year of treatment, flown to his owner's California ranch, where we saw him for the first time. Seeing this beautiful horse's agony and viewing the radiographs of his destroyed feet, I was moved to telephone the veterinarian who had attended him back East.

'Doctor,' I said, 'it is *inhumane* to keep this horse alive. This is the worst case of founder I have ever seen in a living state, and I think we owe it the horse to persuade the owner to do the humane thing.'

'Doctor Miller,' he replied, 'I felt exactly as you do, but let me tell you something. This is no ordinary horse. This horse wants to live. He *tells* me he wants to live. I've never known a horse like him, and you'll soon know what I mean.'

Arabian horses are a large part of my practice. I know them well and am awed by their tenacity and will to go on, but at that time I would gladly have given an overdose of anaesthesia to that poor beast, had I been asked to.

Within a few weeks, however, I learned what the eastern vet meant. This horse's nobility, his goodness, his willingness, and his desire to live were so special, so obvious, that he had ensnared me into that circle of people who had tried so hard to help him.

I put the horse on a special, low-calorie diet. He had been on large amounts of grain which I felt was worsening the founder condition. I kept him on medications to relieve his pain and reduce the inflammation in his feet. We designed special shoes to help support his deformed hooves. X-ray studies showed the bones in his feet, called the coffin bones, were almost completely disintegrated. Miraculously, as time went by, later X-rays showed that these

111

bones were starting to remineralize. After a year of treatment, the bone density was near normal and the pain was subsiding.

Sheik made it! He has even bred mares. His feet will never be normal. He still wears special shoes, and getting up is difficult, but once up he is turned out to pasture and running about with his mane and tail streaming, his lofty gait, his steel-grey coat gleaming, his nostrils flaring, his big, dark, intelligent eyes dominating his classical head, he is the horse painters of every age have immortalized. I love this horse. Few humans have the qualities of character he possesses. Not only brave and beautiful and intelligent, he also has great kindness and affection.

Chapter 18

The first motion picture set I ever saw was for a movie called *Home From the Hills*, a major production starring Robert Mitchum and George Hamilton. The director was Vincente Minnelli, and I don't know if he was still married to Judy Garland at that time, but his thirteen-year-old daughter, Liza Minnelli, hung around the set mooning over Mr Hamilton.

The studio had called me, even though I was nearly seventy miles away, because they had heard I worked with wild animals.

'We need you to anaesthetize a five-hundred-and-thirty-five-pound European wild boar for a hunting scene,' the studio had explained. 'It's for a scene in which the boar has just been shot. Then we'll have some other animals to be anaesthetized too. The boar is supposed to kill a few dogs.'

Debby and I drove to Culver City before dawn. My routine calls would have to be made after I got back in the evening, and I didn't know when I agreed to work on the picture that I would have to return every day for a week. I was yet to be introduced to the incredible slowness and tedium of motion-picture making.

The dog scene came first. I anaesthetized a hound with pentobarbital, a long-lasting anaesthetic. Then the special effects men went to work with the clay and paints and the viscera of a real lamb, and in an hour they had produced an apparently eviscerated dog.

'How does it look, Doctor?' Mr Minnelli asked.

'Well,' I said, 'it's incredibly realistic, but it is anatomically incorrect.'

'What do you mean?' said Minnelli.

'You see, the rumen is hanging out of the wound. Dogs don't have a rumen as sheep do. They should have used the intestines, because the intestines of all animals look pretty much alike. But more important, the viscera are coming from a simulated wound in the thorax – the chest. The digestive viscera should be coming from an abdominal wound. The chest contains only the heart and lungs.'

'Nobody will know the difference,' said Mr Minnelli. 'There aren't that many vets around, and most of them are too busy to go to the movies. We'll use the dog as it is. He looks good.'

'Wait a minute,' I protested. 'There are a lot of people besides veterinarians who know that abdominal viscera shouldn't be hanging out of a chest wound. All doctors would know, and nurses and farmers and butchers and anybody who dissected a frog in high school biology.'

'*I* don't know the difference,' said the director, and the scene was filmed. However, when I saw the finished movie the scene had not been used. I wondered if some editor had suddenly sat up and said, 'Wait a moment, that dog's digestive tract is protruding from a thoracic wound!

Anaesthetizing the boar would have been an easy job today with modern tranquillizing and immobilizing drugs, but with nothing to depend on but barbiturate anaesthetics, which must be injected directly into a vein, I had a real problem. Moreover, the filming was monitored by SPCA officials, and if the boar inadvertently died as a result of drug overdose, they would not permit the scene to be used in the movie. A dead swine that really was dead was unacceptable realism.

The big black boar was put into a chute made of wooden planks. I attempted to inject one of his ear veins, but he was just too wild and vicious to handle. I put a rake handle under his chin in order to elevate his head. He bit the rake handle cleanly in half. I made a mental note to avoid getting my fingers between his huge gleaming tusks.

Finally I sedated the big boar with a combination of narcotic drugs injected into his ham muscles. Then I put a short large needle into his flank and passed a long, slender, blunt needle through it, into his abdomen. I could now do an intra-peritoneal injection. I calculated the dose of sodium pentothal approximately necessary to anaesthetize the boar and injected it into his abdomen. This is an inexact and precarious way to knock out an animal this size, but I had no choice. I had repeatedly tried to inject an ear vein without success, and no other vein was accessible in the boar, unless I were willing to sacrifice an arm.

If I gave too much anaesthetic, the boar could die. Fat animals like swine store barbiturates in their fat and detoxify very slowly, often sleeping for hours or even days. If I gave too little anaesthetic the boar would be insufficiently anaesthetized. He had to look dead without being dead.

Luck was with me. After I gave the injection, the boar was released from the chute. He trotted out into a clearing where the death scene was to be filmed. Then, abruptly, he pitched over on his side, kicked a few times, and was still. 'Quick,' I implored. 'Shoot the scene now. I don't dare give him any more drug.'

The scene was shot, the boar lying motionless except for one upper leg which kept vibrating. A thin wire was used to tie the leg down. When I saw the movie I was able to see the wire, but I'm sure that I was the only one aware of its existence. The scene was shot several times. Then my agony began. I worried that the boar wouldn't wake up. I covered him with blankets, turned him every half hour, and mumbled incantations over him. When I saw signs of the anaesthetic's lightening, I finally went home with my tired wife.

The studio called the next day to tell me that the boar was fine and that Mr Minnelli wanted to talk to me.

'You know how that boar trotted out of the chute and then, bam, fell over on its side?' he asked.

'Yes.'

'Well, I want to duplicate that scene and use it in the movie. It will look just like the boar is shot.'

'I can't do that,' I explained.

'Why not?'

'Because it was a freak situation that he went down that way. I could use the same dose in the same animal the same way, and the chances are he'd never fall down that way again.'

'I know you can do it, Doctor. Be here tomorrow at 6 a.m.'

Debby wisely decided to stay home the next day while I returned to the Culver City studio.

'The SPCA won't let us use the same boar,' I was told.

'Good idea,' I said.

'So we have another boar for you. He's about a hundred pounds smaller, but he's much wilder.'

Using the same technique, I attempted to duplicate the previous day's achievement, but this boar insisted on falling in slow motion. He slowly sagged to the ground while Minnelli fumed and fussed and muttered in exasperation. Repeatedly I would lift the drugged boar to a standing position and then watch him in slow motion spraddle his legs out and sink to the ground. Meanwhile, the cameras kept grinding, in hope that the boar would fall on his side. I wondered how much it cost to keep the huge crowd of technicians on hand and the cameras filming while we waited and the sleepy boar in the centre of the clearing slowly and repeatedly sank downward at an almost imperceptible rate.

'Lift him up again,' Mr Minnelli ordered. He sat peering through the camera, his lower lip nervously twitching. But he never lost his composure or his determination.

'Mr Minnelli,' I begged, as the sun went down, 'I have to go back to Thousand Oaks. I have patients to see. I'll be up half the night.'

'Quiet!' some of the studio workers implored. 'We're on Golden Time!' Apparently the union rules were double salary after so many hours, and the crew was enjoying this benefit by now.

At long last, out of sheer weariness, I think, the boar flopped over on his side and snored mightily while the director gloated, 'I got it! I got it!' I can't recall seeing that scene in the finished movie, so it too may have ended up on the cutting-room floor.

Chapter 19

Ralph Nader has not yet done anything about horse traders, but horse trading is a fertile, everyday field for the defenders of consumers' rights. Equine practitioners are aware that unscrupulous dealers sell horses to unskilled riders and children. Unsound and overpriced horses are sold to unsuspecting buyers under conditions that, if some other commodity were involved, would result in actions involving the Better Business Bureau, the Chamber of Commerce, the Office of Consumer Affairs, and the Bunko Squad.

In the old days, every man was some sort of horseman. The rule of the game in horse trading was *caveat emptor*. Today, the buyer is frequently a middle-class citizen who has never been close to a horse. He is usually buying an animal for his child and is easy pickings for a skilled horse trader. An experienced business or professional man is especially vulnerable to a savvy horse trader. The more shrewd, urbane, and experienced the purchaser is, the better he is as a mark. This kind of buyer cannot believe that the simple country boy he is dealing with would ever tell a lie. ('Shucks! He's too dumb to try to cheat me!')

I made an appointment to see the horse Dennis Walker was planning to buy. I had not met Mr Walker, but he sounded like a decent chap, the father of two boys, aged six and nine.

'This horse is a registered Morgan, and Buck Noonan says he'll be perfect for me and the two boys to learn to ride on.'

'Oh! Oh!' I thought. Buck Noonan, since passed on to the great corral in the sky, was a notorious local horse trader – a glib, amiable cowboy type. He enchanted the city white-collar gentlemen, who confused him with the pure-of-heart heroes in the western films of their childhood years.

'The only reason I'm having a vet check the horse is because he has a problem with one leg,' said Dennis.

'I'll bet!' I thought.

I arrived at the Crooked B ranch (an apt name) before the Walker family. It was early Saturday morning. Two young men were trimming horses' feet.

'Good morning!' I greeted them and explained my mission.

'Oh, yeah,' one called Red said. 'Well, that's the horse

117

over there – the big sorrel with the halter on.'

The corral held about a dozen geldings. These were not California horses. They were all big, raw-boned, hairy-legged, Roman-nosed, and shaggy. They looked like recent imports from northern ranges – Montana maybe. Somewhere up north.

One horse wore a cheap, tattered sale halter. The lead rope hung down to his knees. He looked about twelve years old, and four different brands decorated his hips. He was barefoot, and a mass of proud flesh, painted black, protruded from an old wound on his left hind pastern.

To an experienced horseman, the whole story was obvious. Here was a rank bronc horse from the northern range country. Hard to catch. That's why the halter. Probably hurt a few cowboys and was sold from ranch to ranch. Finally, a barbed-wire cut, doctored cowboy-fashion with 'smear-62,' the old black, government formula. Then, sent south with a truckload of other culled horses. ('Maybe we can unload him in California.') It was a familiar situation.

I caught the horse with difficulty despite the halter. Leading him through the gate was even more difficult. He acted as though he had never seen a gate before.

I cautiously checked him over. When I reached down to examine the injured left hind leg, he cow-kicked at me viciously.

At this point Mr Walker drove up with his two sons. 'What do you think of him?' he asked brightly.

'Well,' I said, 'I thought you said he was a registered Morgan.'

'He is,' Dennis responded. 'They all are. They came down from a ranch near the Canadian border. I've seen the registration papers.'

I bit my lip. 'You know, this is a big, rough, old range horse. If your boys get near his hind end, they might get their heads kicked off.'

'Yes, Buck told us that,' he happily agreed. 'Buck says that a couple of weeks of love and grain and carrots will make him gentle as a lamb.'

'Have you ridden him?' I asked.

'Oh no. He's been out to pasture for almost a year because of his bad leg. Buck says not to ride him until the leg is fixed. That's why I called you. I have to know how much it will cost to fix the leg.'

'Too much, I think,' I answered. 'It will take surgery, and it may cost a hundred dollars, maybe twice that. There'll be a lot of aftercare too. It would be better to start with a sound horse.'

'Oh, but Buck prepared me for that! That's why he's letting me have him so cheap. Where else could I get a registered Morgan for four hundred dollars?'

I could not compete with Buck.

'I'd like to see someone ride him. That's the only way I can fully evaluate him.'

Dennis asked Red if he would ride the horse for me. 'Nope. Can't ride him unless Buck says to, an' he's not here!'

'Then,' I said with satisfaction, 'I'll be unable to complete my examination. I'm going home.'

'Wait!' Red called. He thought a minute and then said, 'Okay, I'll ride him.' Then he turned to his co-worker and ordered, 'Get me that old Heiser saddle.'

I grinned happily while the boys gingerly eased an old bronc saddle on the gelding. Mr Walker was oblivious of the drama about to unfold. If I could get Red bucked off, or could at least create a little spectacle, perhaps Dennis Walker would be shocked into forgetting about the horse.

Red's knuckles were white as he eased up in the saddle. The horse's back was humped as Red cautiously eased him out.

'Move him out!' I yelled. 'Let's see him go!'

Red ignored me and soon skilfully had the horse moving. 'Lope him!' I demanded. 'Kick him out.'

Red kept the horse in a trot until finally the hump was gone from its back. Then Red pushed him into a canter. Alas! The horse was sound, proud flesh and all!

Red pulled up in front of me and smiled maliciously. 'Satisfied?' he asked. He stepped down and said, 'That leg doesn't bother him a bit, does it?'

'May I ride him now?' asked Dennis naively.

Red considered for a moment, and then he made his mistake. 'I guess so,' He answered. 'He's all right.'

Dennis cheerfully mounted. I knew he was going to get dumped. 'Better now, before he buys the horse, than afterwards,' I thought.

As soon as Dennis gained the saddle he spread both legs and enthusiastically thumped both heels into the gelding's sides.

Whoop! The big horse snapped his head down to the ground and bucked straight up into the air. He came down stiff-legged, but it was too late. Dennis Walker was somersaulting through the air. As the horse came up on its second jump, the cantle of the saddle caught Dennis in the middle of his back and spun him backwards. He hit the ground with his left temple.

'A sickening thud,' I thought as I ran forward. 'Now I know what a "sickening thud" is!'

Dennis Walker was a big man, and it took the three of us to hold him down. Every time we released him he staggered to his feet and then fell again. Concussion. Loss of balance. Confused.

I looked up at Red. Red was white. 'Call an ambulance,' I suggested.

'There's a doctor closer,' he said. 'We'll take him.'

Dennis's wife came for the boys, and Dennis was taken to the doctor. I was worried about him. I felt guilty, too. I had known he would be bucked off. Why didn't I stop him?

As soon as my calls were completed, I phoned Mrs Walker.

'He's fine,' she reassured me. 'The X-rays showed no fracture. He has a concussion and has to stay in the hospital, but they said they weren't too worried.'

I phoned again on Monday. Dennis answered the phone.

'Oh, hi, Dr Miller,' he said brightly. 'I'm home again. I'm

fine! Had a brain concussion. They said to stay in bed a few days and take it easy. I appreciate your calling.'

'I sure felt bad about what happened,' I said. 'I was pretty sure that horse was a bucker. That's why I wanted Red to ride him.'

'Is that so? Hey, listen, while we are talking about the horse, when can you do the surgery?'

'What surgery?'

'On his leg. I bought him and have him here at the house. When do you want to operate on his leg?'

It wasn't long before I was calling on another purchaser of his first horse. 'I'll get him,' said Mr Chapin. I had just arrived at the comfortable Chapin home, located on a bluff in the Malibu area, overlooking the sea.

'He has this rash,' said Mr Chapin, as he led the young gelding up to me. After examining the horse, I explained, 'It's just an allergic dermatitis, probably due to fly bites. Nothing serious. I'll give him an injection and leave some medication for you to apply to the lesions. Then, if you'll use a fly repellent spray every morning, perhaps it will solve the problem.

'Good,' smiled Mr Chapin. 'And then will he stop bucking?'

'Bucking?'

'Yes! That's why I called you. I bought the horse for my twelve-year-old daughter, and every time she gets on him he bucks her off. I thought that the rash was making him irritable.'

'Not at all,' I said. 'He's bucking because he's a green colt. He has to be green. He's only two years old.'

'But,' protested Mr. Chapin, 'that's not possible! Mr Noonan said that he was seven years old, gentle, and had been owned by another little girl.'

'Oh, oh!' I said. Buck Noonan had struck again.

'Look,' I said. 'This horse has a two-year-old mouth. He's a baby – a green colt! You have him trained by a professional horse trainer, and I think he'll make a good horse for your daughter. He's a nice looking colt.'

Mr Chapin thanked me. 'I don't know anything about horses,' he said. 'Yesterday, as I watched through the kitchen window, Carol got on the horse, and when he bucked her off, her foot got stuck through the stirrup. He ran off dragging her by one leg, and it's a good thing her boot came off and she came loose. She wasn't seriously hurt. She could have been really injured.'

'She could have been killed,' I said.

As I drove home over the winding mountain roads that connect Malibu with the Conejo Valley, I tried to absorb the rugged scene. The chapparal was blooming, and a variety of lovely flowers contrasted with the harshness of the surrounding brush and rimrock, but I was too upset to enjoy the scenery fully. What kind of man would sell a child an unbroken and dangerous horse? If the child had been killed, I wondered if a jury would have convicted Buck Noonan of manslaughter.

About two weeks later, George Turner called me. The Turners were good clients, a nice family with two teen-aged daughters. They owned several dogs and cats and were frequent visitors at our clinic. The girls both took riding lessons and were eagerly looking forward to owning horses of their own.

'I'd like you to see the horses I bought,' said George Turner. 'The stallion will have to be castrated.'

'You bought a stallion?' I asked.

'Yes! We bought a stallion and a mare. They are mustangs, and the man who caught them and sold them to us said to have the stallion castrated as soon as possible.'

'What do you mean "caught them"?' I inquired. 'Are these wild horses?'

'Yes,' said George. 'He trapped them in the desert. He delivered them this morning. We built a temporary corral by nailing boards to our oak trees, and he backed up a truck and had them jump out of the back end. They're in the corral now. When can you do the surgery?'

'Wait a minute,' I said. 'Let me get this straight. You bought two wild horses for your daughters to ride? They're unbroken mustangs recently caught in the wild?'

'Yes,' said George Turner. 'Buck said that if we fed them carrots and grain for two weeks, they'd be as gentle as kittens and safe for the girls to ride, especially if we castrated the stallion.'

'Buck?' I said. 'Buck Noonan?'

'Yes! Do you know him? Terrific guy! Real cowboy!'

'Listen,' I said. 'I'm going to drop by your place this afternoon. I want to see these horses. Then I'll call you tonight, and we can discuss the surgery.'

When I arrived at the Turner residence, nobody was home except for the family dogs, who knew me. There, behind the house, in a makeshift pen were two small grey horses. I peered through the fence at them. The larger of the two was a stallion, a broomtail, a true mustang. Small and wiry, his long matted tail reached the ground. He was snorting and frightened and cringed in a corner. I judged him to be about seven years of age.

The mare was much older. Tiny and scared. I glimpsed her long yellow teeth as she laid back both ears and charged toward me, whirling as she reached the fence and lashing back with her hind feet, splintering one of the boards. Buck Noonan had sold the naive and trusting George Turner a couple of wild horses for his daughters to ride.

I telephoned later that evening. 'Have you paid for those horses?' I asked. George told me that he had paid Buck half of the agreed upon amount, the balance due in two weeks.

'Mr Turner,' I said, 'You do not want those horses. You phone Buck Noonan and tell him that you want him to return your money and to remove those horses from your property at once.'

The next day George Turner called me and said, 'Doctor Miller, we have always trusted you and had confidence in you as a veterinarian, but we are very disappointed in you as a horse doctor. I called Buck Noonan and told him what you said, and he explained to me that you were simply afraid to handle that stallion. Not that I blame you. Anyway, Buck is coming out this evening with his own vet, a man who isn't afraid of horses, and he will geld the stallion.'

I was deeply hurt. I liked the Turners and was genuinely concerned for their daughters' safety. I had even made a house call at no charge to verify the situation. I had lost the confidence of a client with whom I had had genuine rapport. Worst of all, my ego was damaged. I have always taken great pride in my ability to handle difficult horses. I still do. But back in those days, my pride was mixed with youthful masculine ego. I was offended that George Turner thought my reason for advising him not to keep the horses was fear.

'George!' I said. 'If you keep those horses, it will end in tragedy.'

'What kind of tragedy?' he asked.

'I don't know,' I said. 'But it *will* end in some kind of tragedy.'

'Doctor Miller,' George said confidently, 'don't worry about it. Buck and his vet know how to handle horses of this kind.'

The next morning George Turner telephoned me. 'Doctor Miller,' he said, his voice quavering. 'I owe you an apology.'

'What happened?' I asked.

'Buck came out last night with his own vet. They roped the stallion and wrapped the rope around a branch. I never saw an animal scream and fight like that in my life. It was awful. The stallion was choking and he fell down, kicking. The vet tried to get an injection into him, but he never was able to. And then, suddenly, the horse stopped struggling. He was dead, Doctor Miller. He died there right in front of my entire family. I have never experienced anything like it. I told Buck to load the mare back onto his truck and to get off my place and never return, and I made him return my deposit. I wish I had listened to you. I don't think my girls will ever forget the horror of seeing that horse die.'

Chapter 20

Once I had opened an office, I needed an assistant to run it. I placed an ad in the local newspaper, and the first person to answer it was Mrs Mary Tuttle. When she introduced herself (this was more than a quarter century ago, remember), she curtsied, and in that simple, old-fashioned gesture she revealed everything about her sturdy, old-fashioned up-bringing: her good character, her reliability, and her sense of propriety. Mary and Debby were all the staff I had in those days.

'Now that we have an office, we need a cat,' Debby said. Many animal hospitals kept a cat as a mascot and as an occasional blood donor if a patient needed a transfusion.

Debby was sitting at the desk with a newly neutered tom-cat on her lap. She was commiserating with him over his loss and explaining to him his new role in life as a home-loving companion. 'We need a cat of our own,' she said.

'Right,' I agreed. 'We'll watch for a suitable kitten.'

Unwanted kittens or, for that matter, animals of all kinds are abundantly available to animal hospitals. Nearly all such places have residents that were unwanted pets, and if you go to the home of a veterinarian or any employee of a veterinary hospital, you are sure to see adopted animals that were abandoned patients.

Thus it was that a lost kitten was presented to us one day. She was a tiny tri-coloured calico kitten – white and black and red – and although she had the face of a feline, her body more resembled that of a hare. She was promptly named Harvey the Rabbit.

Harvey apparently belonged to a strain of cats indigenous to the Conejo Valley that had short forelegs, long hind legs, and a little fuzzy ball of a tail, just like that of a cottontail rabbit. Legend had it that these cats were all descended from a Jungleland bobcat that was crossbred with a domestic cat. I never believed that story. Wild bobcats are abundant in southern California, and many of them have been captured as kittens and brought up as pets. Moreover, the bobcat will crossbreed with the domestic cat, but I think that our Conejo Valley short-tailed cats were simply a mutation similar to the one that produced the Manx breed. Anyway, these rabbity-looking cats were common in our community until the increasing influx of new residents in the sixties, moving in with cats of more conventional conformation, genetically obliterated the tail-less Conejo Valley strain.

Spayed, vaccinated, and well-fed, Harvey grew into the perfect office mascot. Her favourite resting place was on the fireplace mantel in our reception room where she would sleep in a crouched position with her face buried between her paws. Awakening, she startled many clients who thought she was a decorative piece of statuary. She was a friendly and inquisitive cat, and many of our clients were fascinated by her personality and her unusual appearance. There were people who would stop by to visit her and bring her treats, especially at Christmas time. 'Where's Harvey?' many clients would want to know if she wasn't in the front room when they came in.

Harvey ignored other cats, but she personally had to greet every dog that came into the clinic. She would leap down from the mantel and regally make her way to the canine visitor. Harvey enjoyed a suicidal game with large dogs, batting at their tails. We often feared that this pastime would eventually lead to a disaster, but the dogs seemed to know that they were on her turf, and most were too filled with anxiety when in our waiting room to be concerned about the antics of the ridiculous-looking cat boxing with their tails.

Although she was never trained to do so, Harvey would retrieve like a dog. A roll of gauze, thrown like a ball, would be pursued across the floor with much skidding and sliding and immediately brought back and dropped at the thrower's feet. She never tired of this game and would play it as long as one would participate.

A Newcomers Club formed in town, and Debby and I joined it because it enabled us to meet other young couples. The meetings were held monthly, rotating through the members' homes and at one of these meetings our hostess said, 'Doc, we have a kitten that looks like a rabbit, and we'd like to bring it in Monday for its shots.' They then produced a kitten, about six months of age, that, except for being two-thirds the size of Harvey, was absolutely identical to our cat. The only difference was that Harvey had a black right ear, and this cat's right ear was white. Other than that, it looked like Harvey, including the distribution of black and red markings on a white background, the rabbitlike legs, and the cotton-ball tail.

Debby and I marvelled at the similarity and explained the coincidence to the kitten's owners. We agreed the two cats had to be closely related even though Harvey was several years older.

I had an idea. I offered to take the cat back to the clinic with me. 'We'll vaccinate her and keep her over the weekend, and you can pick her up on Monday,' I suggested. Finding a Harvey duplicate was an opportunity too unusual not to take advantage of. We took the kitten with us and dyed the right ear with ink.

Early Monday morning I hid Harvey in a cage in the back room and put the new kitten on the floor of the examining room. When Mary came in I busied myself at my desk.

'Good morning, Doctor Miller,' Mary called out.

'Morning, Mary,' I responded.

'Good morning, Harvey,' Mary said next. Then, there was a long silence.

'Doctor Miller?'

'Yes?'

'Harvey is shrinking!'

'What's that?'

'Harvey is *shrinking*!'

'That right?' I responded vaguely. 'Well, if she's losing weight, just feed her a little more.'

'I don't mean that she's losing weight!' Mary exploded. 'I

mean she's shrinking! She's getting smaller!'

'Now Mary,' I soothed her. 'Harvey's never been a big cat. You're just used to seeing all those lions and tigers and so on coming in here.'

'Doctor Miller,' Mary insisted, thrusting 'Harvey' at me, 'look at her! She's getting smaller. How is this possible?'

I peered at 'Harvey' and took the kitten from her and speculatively weighed it in my hands.

'I believe you're right,' I said. 'Harvey *is* getting smaller. This is interesting.'

'But how can it be?' Mary demanded with great concern. 'What's going on?'

'Well,' I mused, 'I'm not sure. We must have something unusual here. Perhaps she got into one of our medicine cabinets, and we are seeing some kind of drug side-effect. Or maybe she's been hanging around the X-ray machine. I saw this movie last year called *The Incredible Shrinking Man*. A guy gets exposed to some kind of radiation, and one day he notices his clothes are too big, and when he stands next to his wife, he realizes she is suddenly taller than he is, so he. . .'

'Doctor Miller!' Mary squinted at me suspiciously and raised a threatening finger.

'Tell you what I'll do,' I went on. 'I'll give her an injection of a growth hormone, and I'll bet that by tomorrow she'll be back up to normal size.'

But Mary was too sharp for that. 'Doctor Miller,' she said, 'I don't know how it's possible, but this can't be Harvey! Where in the world did you ever find this cat, and where is the real Harvey?'

I was fortunate to have found Mary to run the office, since the practice continued to grow to the point where I was carrying a staggering work load, caring for great numbers of pets, livestock, horses, and wild animals, and on call every night of the week. I needed more help badly.

One day a tall, gangling, young crew-cut veterinarian visited me. His name was Bob Kind. A Kansas farm boy, he had served a couple of years as a military veterinarian after finishing his education and was now employed in a Los Angeles pet practice. He was looking for a permanent location, and the Conejo Valley looked promising to him.

We made arrangements to meet at a restaurant at a halfway point between Los Angeles and Thousand Oaks so that we could meet each other's wives and get better acquainted.

Debby is an astute judge of character, and I told her that if she approved of the Kinds as future associates to signal me by saying to me, 'Oh! Did you remember to return Mrs Johnson's call?'

If she disapproved of the Kinds, she would simply remain silent, and I would avoid making any commitments at that time.

We met, sat down to dinner, and had barely started our salads when Debby said, 'Oh! Did you remember to return Mrs Johnson's call before we left town?'

I looked at her in amazement because Debby rarely makes decisions quickly. She explained later that she promptly decided that the Kinds were good people.

'Yes,' I answered, 'I called her.' Then we started to discuss the future with Bob and Mary Lee Kind.

Accepting Dr Bob Kind as an associate, and eventually as a partner, was one of the best decisions I ever made, because this tall, gentle, honest man with whom I've never had a quarrel or even a major difference of opinion is more to me than a professional colleague and a business partner. He is a trusted friend.

Bob is about six-and-a-half feet tall, and although he was three years out of veterinary school and had been an Air Force officer, he looked very youthful. One morning a client came in with a dog. This gentleman was the basketball coach for a college that had recently opened in Thousand Oaks. As we spoke, Bob Kind walked through the room. The coach looked at Bob, stopped speaking abruptly, and then, after Bob had left the room, asked excitedly, 'Hey! Who is that kid? I want him for my team!'

'That kid,' I explained, 'is Dr Kind, my new associate. He played basketball in college, but that's all behind him today.'

The coach looked crestfallen. His team's performance was not impressive that year. If Bob had played for him, perhaps the team would have done better.

One of my best accounts in those days was Don Swanson. Don was a well-to-do, owned several fine horses and a bunch of dogs and cats. He was a valued client who expected and received prompt and skilful service. While not exactly demanding, Mr Swanson was precise in his requests for service. I was concerned that he might not accept my new associate, but would demand that I personally cater to his animals. Bob Kind attended his dogs and horses for a couple of months until, one day, Mary confided in me.

'Mr Swanson requested that, whenever possible, Doctor Kind be scheduled to see his animals. He said that he and Mrs Swanson really respected Doctor Miller, but they found Doctor Kind to be deliberate, just as they are. They asked me not to tell you, but asked if, whenever possible, they could see Doctor Kind. I knew you wouldn't be offended and would be relieved to know that they like him.'

I was as pleased at the news as I was surprised. Above all, I was relieved. My new associate had been accepted.

Chapter 21

Ike was the foreman of a cattle ranch near Thousand Oaks. While chatting with him as I cleaned up my equipment after treating a cow, a small nondescript mongrel wandered lazily out of the barn in to the fading afternoon sunlight. I noted a ragged scar on the dog's left side, curving from the lumbar area to the flank.

'That's a nasty scar,' I said to the dog. 'What did you tangle with?'

The dog didn't answer, but Ike did. 'We never did find out, Doc. He just came acrawlin' home one day with this here big hole in his side and with all his intestine ahangin' out of it. No tellin' how far he'd come. He was a mess!'

I studied the old injury with renewed interest. It was zig-zagged and thickened with scar tissue. I knew that I had not repaired that wound, so I asked if the veterinarian who had formerly served the ranch had done so.

'Heck, no! I wouldn't spend no money on that two-bit dog. I jest brushed off the grass and dirt and stuffed his guts back in and pulled the skin back together with five or six of them spring-clip clothespins.'

I stared at Ike for a while. 'What happened?'

'Oh, he lay curled up in the barn for a week or so. Wouldn't eat. Wouldn't get up, I kept expectin' him to die. Then one day he came awalkin' slow and awaggin' his tail. He sure looked comical with all those clothespins stickin' out from his side.'

I digested this, and asked. 'You must have loaded him up with penicillin, huh?'

'Heck, no Doc. I figured he was goin' to die anyway. I'da put him out of his misery, but the old lady wanted me to try.'

After further pondering, I decided that the wound had not penetrated the abdominal cavity. What Ike thought was intestine must have been subcutaneous tissue and fat.

'I don't think that was intestines hanging out, Ike,' I suggested. 'It was probably torn muscle, fat, and tissue.'

Ike looked offended. 'Doc, I done a lot of butcherin'. I know intestine when I see it. It was ahangin' out, several feet; long old tubes strung together with a curtain with veins in it. It was intestine. I jest brushed off the grass and all the dirt, and stuffed 'er back in. Then I put the clothespins on!'

I don't have a lot of trouble with postoperative infection, but every time I've experienced one, I've winced and thought about Ike and that dog.

The medical ingenuity of the American stockman never ceases to amaze me. I recall the cowboy who replaced a cow's prolapsed uterus out on the range and then sutured the vulva closed with his pocket knife and hairs from his horse's tail. I think of the rancher who laced together a gaping wound in a horse's shoulder, using baling wire and a leather punch.

Stockmen have done caesarean sections and rumenotomies and have fixed fractures. But Ike's clothespin operation takes the cake. I don't know how that dog survived the shock, avoided infection, and stood up to the post-traumatic stress, but I'm willing to bet that if that repair had been attempted in a sparkling operating room, with sterilized instruments, a gloved and gowned surgeon, and all the other amenities of modern medicine, the dog would have died on the table.

Veterinarians must still perform operations in the barnyard or even out on the range. Mostly, though, we perform surgery in modern, antiseptic facilities.

Tony Gentry had a pony farm. One of his ponies suffered an intestinal blockage, and for four days I had been trying to relieve the little horse's colic, without success. 'He's weakening,' I explained to Tony, 'and I'm afraid that the only chance he has is for us to open him up. He's small enough to fit on a small-animal operating table in our hospital, so let's do him there.'

The pony was moved to our clinic, anaesthetized,

hooked up to intravenous fluids, and prepared for abdominal surgery. Bob and I scrubbed and donned cap, mask, gowns, and gloves while an assistant prepared the pony's abdomen. The 'prepped' belly was then covered with sterile drapes, and the operation began. The procedure took a couple of hours, during which we successfully opened the abdomen, relieved the obstruction, and then carefully closed the incision with multiple layers of suturing. After the pony woke up, we jubilantly helped it into a trailer and watched Tony take it home.

Two days later, I was attending a Lion's Club luncheon, when a waitress came in and called, 'Doctor Miller, you have an emergency call.'

It was Tony Gentry.

'There's something hanging out of the incision, Doc,' he said. 'Looks like guts or something, and it's sticking out maybe six inches.'

I raced to Tony's place in Newbury Park. When I arrived, the man's face was a portrait of despair. 'Put him down, Doc,' he implored. 'Let's end it!'

The pony was dejectedly standing in the stall. While I drove from the luncheon, the incision had completely opened up, and the poor creature was standing in his own intestines. They were wrapped around his legs and covered with mud and manure.

'Just put him down, Doc. We can't take any more!'

'Not on your life,' I said. 'Not after all the work we did to try to save him. I'm not going to put him down!'

I anaesthetized the pony and asked for a garden hose and some bed sheets. The intestine was washed off as best we could, and the sheets were placed under it to keep it as clean as possible. Then, after hastily washing my hands, I stuffed everything back into the abdomen, flicking away the larger clods of dirt and manure as I did so. Then I poured an entire bottle of antibiotic solution into the abdominal cavity. After the last of it gurgled in, I hastily sewed the belly closed.

The pony lived and to the best of my knowledge is still

alive at a very advanced age. So, you see, crude barnyard surgery is sometimes effective. As another example, I might cite the case of Roy Morrison's cow.

Bob Kind performed a caesarean section on one of Morrison's beef cows. The patient recovered nicely from what is a routine operation in a country veterinary practice.

Several days after the operation the owner called Bob. 'That cow has a huge swelling under the incision,' he explained. 'We've got her roped and tied to an oak tree.'

It was nearly dark when Bob arrived. The cow then was stretched out, her head tied to the tree, and her hind feet to the bumper of Bob's car. She was so debilitated that, rather than giving her a general anaesthetic, Bob opened the incision under local anaesthesia. The inner layers of the belly wall had given way. Fortunately the skin sutures had held, but a length of black gangrenous intestine filled the swelling on the cow's belly. The hernia had strangulated, and the blood supply being squeezed off, the intestine had become gangrenous. Working alone while Mr Morrison held a flashlight, my partner removed eight feet of gangrenous intestine, and then anastomosed the viable portion of the gut, sewing the cut ends of the healthy intestine end-to-end to re-establish the continuity of the intestinal tract. He then closed the abdominal wall.

'Think she'll make it?' I asked the next day as Bob told me of his operation in the dark.

'Probably dead already,' Bob observed pessimistically.

Several months later I was examining the entire Morrison herd for pregnancy. Most of the cows were in calf, and they all looked fat and healthy. We were down to the last few head in the herd when an emaciated cow entered the examining chute. I lubricated my gloved arm and pushed it into the rectum. Just below the rectum, I could feel the uterus and ovaries of the cow. The organs filled my hand. No pregnancy here.

'No wonder,' I said. 'She's in terrible shape! What's wrong with her?'

Roy Morrison's eyebrows went up. 'Why, that's "Old

Miracle",' he protested, 'and she looks great! You should have seen her a few weeks ago.'

'Old Miracle?' I asked.

'Sure!' said the rancher. 'That's the cow your partner opened up and cut out eight feet of gut. Why, I never saw or heard of anything like it. That was a miracle, and that cow has a home on my ranch for the rest of her natural life.'

When the Morrisons sold their ranch to developers and moved to a new place up north, 'Old Miracle' went with them, a living testimonial to a triumph of barnyard surgery.

Chapter 22

I can't remember exactly when Belle Holloway died; sometime during the sixties. I prefer to remember her as she was when she lived: a remarkable woman known as 'the woman who talked to horses.'

Born in the last half of the nineteenth century in a cabin near what is now Thousand Oaks, Belle Holloway spent her entire life in the Conejo Valley. She told me stories of the old days – of riding horseback to Santa Barbara, of the stagecoach that connected Newbury Park (the only community in the Conejo Valley at that time) with the Simi Valley, and of how old-time ranchers used to run hogs on open range to fatten on the native acorns. After the turn of the century, hog cholera destroyed the swine industry. Agriculture in our valley was thereafter limited to grazing cattle and dry-land grain farming.

Livestock, especially horses, was Belle's life. She was a

marvellous hand with horses and could handle the toughest of them. Even after a total mastectomy, which practically incapacitated one arm, she was a wizard at loading, breaking, and gentling young horses. By the time I moved into her area, Belle Holloway was operating a successful horse-hauling business. Her brown trucks and trailers were a familiar sight on California's highways. Thousands of race-horses commuted the length of the state in them.

A warm, talkative, jovial woman, and a grandmother, Belle personally drove a big semi-rig loaded with valuable horses. A two-way public address system connected the trailer to the cab. In those pre-tranquilliser days, if Belle heard a horse acting up in the back while she was speeding down the road, she would pick up her microphone and talk to the horse, calming and soothing it. When I think of Belle, I picture her driving that big rig down the highway, her blue-grey granny's head peering over the wheel, microphone in hand, talking to the horses.

Belle was of the old school, a genuine country woman. Once when she made an appointment with me to geld some colts, she warned, 'Doc, you know I checked with the almanac, and the sign ain't right, but I don't suppose you believe in that.'

I told her, 'Belle, if I waited until the sign was right, I'd have to do all my gelding on one day, and that would be inconvenient. Anyway, I haven't lost a colt yet, so I must be doing something right.' We gelded the horses without benefit of the almanac.

Belle fell in with a quackish fellow named Dr Scroggins. He was, she said, a chiropractor who had got into trouble treating people, so now he was treating horses. Scroggins, Belle explained, had two marvellous machines. One of these was a diagnostic machine. A piece of paper with a drop of patient's blood was mailed to Scroggins. The paper was put into the machine, and lo, the diagnosis would come out.

Belle wanted to believe in the machine. She was unschooled, but her common sense caused her to question it. 'Ever heard of a machine like that?' She squinted at me challengingly. 'No,' I confessed, 'but let's test it out. Let's send him a drop of chicken blood, and tell him it's a thoroughbred filly's blood.'

Scroggins's diagnosis soon arrived. The chicken, it seemed, had azoturia, a horse disease. 'Why, I didn't know that chickens got azoturia,' Belle said.

Scroggins's other machine was a therapeutic device which he leased to Belle. Known as the 'black box,' it was a jumble of tubes and electric wires. When plugged in and focused on the patient, it supposedly could cure anything.

Once Belle asked me to examine a 'wobbler' colt. 'Wobblers' results in uncoordination due to a spinal defect. I confirmed the diagnosis, gave a poor prognosis, and said I felt that any specific therapy was probably useless. I suggested pasturing the horse for a year to see if 'tincture of time' would result in improvement. Belle said, 'Well, I'm going to use the box on this colt. It will be a good test.'

The horse was, of course, normal a year later, by my own admission. Soon wobblers were coming to Belle's farm from all over the state. None of them ever improved, but Scroggins's single victory was cited far and wide.

One day Belle brought me a sample of manure and asked me to check it for worms. I prepared a faecal flotation test and allowed her to see the myriad strongyle eggs under the microscope.

'Good,' she said. 'I want you to help me run an experiment. Doc Scroggins says I can worm horses by shining his machine on their hind end. I'm going to use it on this horse, and in a couple of weeks, we'll run another test to see if there are any worms left.'

I agreed to do this, pointing out that, in the interest of science, I would not charge for the lab work.

Eventually, Belle brought in the second faecal specimen. Through the microscope I could see many worm eggs. I moved over to let her look. She peered through the lens for a long time, silently and without changing expression. Finally she straightened up and said, 'Well, that's what I get for messing around with Scroggin's directions. He said to shine it on the hind end for ten minutes a day, and I was afraid it was too strong a dose, so I only gave it five minutes. Looks like five minutes is not enough. Anyway, it takes too long and it's too much trouble. Give me some phenothiazine, Doc!'

Once I treated a huge, stubborn hunter at a stable a half-hour's drive from my office. The animal, a notorious outlaw when getting into a trailer was involved, needed daily treatment for wounds incurred in a trailer-loading accident. The owner liked my suggestion that the horse be moved to Belle Holloway's place, which was just a short distance from my office. The problem was how to transport this big, trailer-shy, and already injured horse.

'Belle can handle it,' I assured the apprehensive owner. I called Belle, suggesting she transport the horse in a van. 'They're all on the road,' she replied. 'I'll pick him up myself in a trailer.'

'Belle,' I said, 'I know you're good at loading horses, but this guy is really bad medicine. I'm not sure you'll be able to load him without a van.'

'Doc,' she answered, 'they can all be loaded. I'll take care of it.'

The next day Belle called. 'That big red horse is at my place if you want to come out and doctor him. You know, Doc, that was the toughest horse to load I ever saw.'

'I warned you,' I chided. 'What happened?'

'Well, I went through my whole repertoire of tricks. I talked to him, I coaxed him, I hypnotized him, but he wouldn't load. I tried the war bridle, and I even used my special secret methods for real bad horses. But you know, I worked for hours, and I couldn't load that horse. Finally, I hate to admit it, but I lost my temper, got out a bull whip, and I beat the hell out of that horse until he finally was *glad* to jump into that trailer!'

Chapter 23

Sometimes it is necessary, for humane reasons, for a veterinarian to destroy a large animal by shooting it. We are trained how to do this properly. The brain of a horse or cow is no larger than a man's fist, and if the bullet is properly placed, death is instantaneous. If, however, the bullet misses the brain, an animal that size may show startlingly little effect from a gunshot wound. In order to locate the brain, we draw an 'X' on the forehead, from the left eye to the right ear, and from the right eye to the left ear. Where the lines intersect, a bullet will enter the brain.

It was midnight. Debby and I were driving back to Thousand Oaks. We had gone into the city to see a show. Far up the highway I could see flashing red lights and flares. I slowed as I approached the scene.

Three Brahman bulls had escaped from a pasture and wandered onto the highway into the path of two trucks. One bull had been killed. Another had been hit but fled up into the mountains. The last had a broken back and was sitting dog fashion, in the middle of the highway.

Unaware of the nature of the accident, I heard a shot fired as I came closer. 'That was a gunshot,' I said to Debby with some concern, and slowed to a crawl. From the confusion of flares and flashing police lights came a second shot. I stopped the car. If the police ahead were involved in a gunfight, I didn't want to come any closer. Then my headlights picked up the figure of a cowboy running toward me, waving me on, and shouting, 'Keep moving! Go on!'

I recognized Harlan Brown, the foreman of the surrounding Triunfo Ranch. 'What's going on, Harlan?' I yelled through the open window.

'Doc!' he exclaimed. 'Just the man we need!'

A third shot sounded up ahead.

'The highway patrol's trying to shoot a crippled bull. I think they need help!'

139

I drove up, got out of the car, and approached an officer holding a .38 special revolver. He had just fired five rounds into the head of the bull from a distance of ten feet. The bull sat, looking pathetically unconcerned, a tiny trickle of blood leaking from one nostril. Several bullet holes were visible in the area of the frontal sinus.

'This here man is our vet,' said Harlan. 'Would you like him to shoot the bull?' The officer looked at me coldly, and then asked Harlan, 'Is this your bull?'

'No sir, he comes from a different ranch.'

'Well, then, I'll shoot the bull,' spoke the law.

With that he took aim and fired again. The bull didn't even flinch.

'Do you want me to shoot him?' I asked.

No answer. Having fired all six rounds from the revolver, the officer turned to another patrolman. 'Give me your magnum, Bill.'

Now armed with a .357 magnum, the patrolman again aimed from a cautious distance. The revolver boomed. The bull still sat there. Then came the unforgettable remark: in disgust, frustration, and embarrassment, the officer bellowed, 'What in hell is wrong with these goddam guns?'

Nobody answered. He turned to me. 'Do *you* want to shoot this bull?'

'Yes.'

'Be careful now!' he warned, handing me the weapon.

I stepped briskly up to the bull, drew an 'X' with lines running from his left ear to his right eye and from his right ear to his left eye, placed the muzzle where the lines of ruffled hair intersected, and pulled the trigger. The bull collapsed, instantaneously dead, his suffering mercifully ended.

I returned the revolver and looked at the officer. 'Did you see how I did it?' I asked him. He nodded dumbly, his mouth hanging open. 'Did you see how I made the cross on his head?'

'Yeah! You're a Catholic, huh Doc?'

*

Only rarely does this taking of life have any comedy associated with it. Ending the life of an animal is the most unpleasant task a veterinarian has to perform. Our training and our instincts are directed towards the preservation of life. Nevertheless, all veterinary practitioners must inevitably perform this service, at all too frequent intervals. We refer to the deed by its technical term: *euthanasia*. Pet owners usually say 'put to sleep.' This is a bit of a risky euphemism because I know of several cases where an owner asked the veterinarian to 'put the animal to sleep,' meaning that they wanted whatever treatment is necessary to be done under general anaesthesia. Misunderstanding, the veterinarian then put the animal to sleep permanently. In order to prevent such a mishap, we always request that the owner or his representative sign a document formally requesting euthanasia.

Horse people usually say 'put him down' when they mean to request euthanasia, and again, this term is sometimes confused with general anaesthesia.

I rarely recommend euthanasia for a patient, even if I know that the case is hopeless and that the animal deserves to be spared unnecessary suffering. Instead, I will say, 'I know what I would do if this were my animal, but that is a decision you must make.' This gives the owner the opportunity of accepting the humane alternative, without being able to accuse me of wanting to kill his animal. The reason I do things this way is because of an incident that occurred shortly after I opened my first little clinic in Thousand Oaks. I had diagnosed terminal cancer in an old spaniel owned by an elderly gentleman. The owner, even after I had explained the suffering the dying dog was experiencing, requested medication to help relieve the pain. He brought the poor animal in each day. I did what I could, but as I saw the progressive wasting of the dog's body and saw that look in his eyes which is characteristic of terminal cancer, I began to feel guilty. I had suggested euthanasia at each visit as an alternative. Finally, I said to the owner, 'Look, you are not being fair to this animal. His

141

condition is hopeless. He is suffering terribly even though he cannot express his feelings, and I think that it is time to do the merciful thing.'

The old man looked at me stonily and said, 'Young man, you're a doctor, and you have knowledge that I do not have, and that is, how to prolong this dog's life and to make his remaining time as comfortable as possible. I came to you to help my dog, not to destroy him. If I wanted to destroy him, I could have left him in a closed garage with the car motor running.'

With that he gathered up the shrunken, emaciated body of his pet and walked out saying, 'I will find a veterinarian who is more interested in fending off death than he is in causing it.'

There is, however, another aspect to this subject. What if the owner wants the animal to be killed, but the veterinarian is personally opposed to it?

Mr Bigelow was a local businessman in his late sixties. He owned a perfectly beautiful Tennessee Walking Horse mare, and it was a common sight to see him riding along the narrow twisting main thoroughfare through Thousand Oaks. The mare was about ten years of age, and covered the ground at the swift and spectacular gait so typical of that breed. 'Goldie' was stabled in a completely enclosed box stall, kept blanketed all year round, and was shod with the heavy built up shoes and elongated feet that many walking horse owners prefer. Usually this exaggerated and unnatural method of shoeing is reserved for show horses. Mr Bigelow did not show his mare, but he kept her shod that way anyway, as a matter of preference.

One evening he called me and asked if I could be at his home to 'take care' of his mare at nine the next morning. The Bigelow home was not far from the little house Debby and I had rented. We had progressed from living in a garage to a small house that flooded every time it rained.

The next morning, when I arrived at the Bigelows', I was surprised to see the Jungleland dead animal truck parked in

142

front. I suddenly realized that I was expected to perform a euthanasia.

'Doctor,' said Mr Bigelow, 'I know that she must be shot if Jungleland is to take her, and I know that shooting is swift and merciful, but I do not want to be here. I would like to pay your fee, and sign any necessary papers, and then I will leave, and you do what is necessary.'

'But why am I doing this?' I asked. I was distressed. The mare was tied to an oak tree nearby and looked perfectly healthy. 'What's wrong with her? Why are we doing this?'

'Doctor, I have a very bad heart condition, I will not be able to ride any longer, and I don't think I have long to live.'

I now noticed how pale and wan Mr Bigelow looked. His complexion was almost grey.

'I want to be sure that Goldie is taken care of before I pass on,' he said.

'But she looks so healthy,' I protested.

'She is,' he agreed. 'She's in perfect condition. That's why I want her put down. Nobody else will take care of her as I have, and I must know that she will never be abused. She has meant a lot to me.'

I looked at the mare, an elegant animal in the prime of her life. Her coat gleamed in the morning light. Her mane and tail were fastidiously groomed.

'Look,' I said, 'I'm a veterinarian. I have a mare of my own and the use of a nice pasture next to my house. Will you give Goldie to me? I will pledge never to sell her and always to give her the best of care.'

'Never,' Bigelow shouted. '*Nobody* will care for her as I have. She is locked in a stall every moment when I'm not riding her. She is kept blanketed, and those special shoes cost a fortune. I know that you wouldn't do those things!'

'That's true,' I argued, 'but you see those things as a kindness, and I don't. I know that Goldie would be happier in a pasture and rid of those blankets and those awful shoes. She doesn't need blankets in this climate. I like Walking Horses, and I'd shoe her natural, and she would enjoy life

143

much more that way. Wouldn't that be better than killing her?'

'No!' Mr Bigelow shouted. 'If you won't do this, I'll call someone who will!' He was flustered and angry, and I suddenly remembered that this man was near death from a bad heart.

'All right!' I weakened, 'I'll do it, but I sure don't feel right about it.'

I was in a dilemma, torn between the wish of a dying man, and my own reluctance to destroy the beautiful mare I had admired so often since I had moved to town. I was also inexperienced and insecure and trying to establish a practice in this little town, and Mr Bigelow was one of the more influential and successful local businessmen.

After Mr Bigelow left, I put his mare down. When I saw her lying on the ground, dead, her eyes glazed, I knew that I had done the wrong thing. I vowed that I would never again take a life if my own conscience was opposed to that action. I have never broken that vow. I have had to end the lives of many hundreds of animals since that morning, but never because the owner wished it done while I was opposed to it.

I saw Mr Bigelow many times after the Jungleland truck hauled Goldie away. The last time I saw him, he looked exactly as he did the morning his mare died. He was thin and grey-faced, but he looked no older even though eleven years had gone by.

Attending to this ultimate responsibility is never easy, but it is especially difficult when the animal is one the veterinarian has treated and grown attached to during the years.

Swampy was a mongrel of unrecognizable ancestry, but a benevolent genius of dogdom. He was a neighbour as well as a patient. Ignoring all leash laws he would visit my house, jump the fence, play tag with my dogs, and then, as dinnertime approached, he would return (over the fence) to his own home.

144

Swampy looked tough. He was a muscular, prick-eared, yellow mongrel with many scars about his alert face. He looked tough, but in reality, Swampy loved all men and all beasts. His heart, like his coat, was of gold. He enjoyed fine health, and most of my professional contacts with him involved preventive medicine and routine physical examinations. As he aged, I was saddened to see that arthritis kept him from jumping into my yard. No other neighbour's dog would have been welcome, but Swampy never dumped over the trash, littered my property, chased the stock, or did anything wrong.

When Swampy was fourteen years old he developed a malignant lung tumour the size of a hen's egg. We operated, removing the diseased portion of the lung. Swampy survived the surgery and made an uneventful recovery. At fifteen years of age, he was still going strong, although quite hard of hearing and a bit doddering. He'd still grin when he came in, wag his tail, and say 'Hi Doc!' Swampy was a favourite with our hospital staff and all of his neighbours. When he was hospitalized, some of his friends sent a bouquet of flowers.

Swampy's master had a job offer in another city, so one day his mistress brought the old dog in to say goodbye to us. I patted the old yellow head and told him I'd miss him. What I didn't tell him was that I was glad he was leaving. I knew Swampy didn't have much time left. I was grateful that I would not be the veterinarian who would, some day soon, have to put Swampy permanently to sleep.

Chapter 24

It was Bob's night on emergency duty when the Bar Jay Stable called about a horse that had been badly cut by barbed wire. It was so good to have an associate to share the emergency case load with. The nights off were a luxury, and we each took alternate Thursdays off. On Saturday we both worked regularly because that was our busiest day. Bob repaired the deep and nasty laceration, and the stable owner told us to bill the owner of the horse, which was being boarded. The bill was never paid. Since I owned the practice at the time, Bob working for me and not yet a partner, I attempted to collect the bill. I called the horse's owner, a Mr Hayes, and learned that the horse had fully recovered and that he was very pleased with Doctor Kind's surgical repair.

'So why don't you pay the bill?' I asked. 'It's been half a year since the call was made.' The owner explained that he had not authorized the stable to put his horse in a barbed-wire enclosure. The injury was therefore the stable's fault, and they should be responsible for the bill. He had given our bills to the stable owner, a Mr Hennesman, who had stated that he had no intention of paying them. Mr Hayes said that he was grateful to us and very sad that we hadn't been paid, but he insisted that Mr Hennesman and not he was responsible for the bill. I suggested that he pay the bill to demonstrate his gratitude, and then come to some sort of an agreement with Mr Hennesman. Hayes said that he wasn't going to do that. It was up to us to get paid by Mr Hennesman, who, unfortunately, had the reputation among veterinarians of not paying his bills.

Eventually I took the case to small claims court, convinced that we had a legally substantial claim against Hayes. I took half a day off to go to the courtroom in Camarillo.

Mr Hayes appeared too, a middle-aged man, nicely

dressed and well-mannered.

To my surprise, the judge ruled in his favour after hearing the case.

'Doctor,' the judge said, 'I sympathize with you. Your associate did a good job, and it hasn't been paid for. However, the verbal contract was made over the telephone with the stable owner, and therefore Mr Hayes is right. He doesn't owe you the fee. Mister Hennesman does.'

'But,' I protested, 'we accepted the call knowing that another person owned the horse and assumed that the owner would appreciate our service and be willing to pay for it.'

'But,' the judge insisted, 'Mister Hayes was never consulted about the matter. The agreement was between Doctor Kind and Mister Hennesman. He is the man whom you must pursue.'

Knowing that to pursue Hennesman was probably futile, I left the courtroom frustrated and sorry I had taken the time to go to court.

As I left the building I passed Mr Hayes. 'I'm sorry, Doctor,' he said, 'sorry you and Doctor Kind got stuck like this, but it is a matter of principle. Hennesman was responsible for my horse's being hurt, and I won't pay his bill!'

'You know,' I said, 'I haven't been in practice a long time, but in the few years I have been, this sort of thing has happened too many times, but it won't happen again. I vow that we'll never again answer an emergency call to see an injured animal unless the owner personally places the call and agrees to be responsible for the charges.'

I knew that I was making an idle threat, because a great percentage of veterinary emergency calls are requested by people who don't own the animal involved. A stray animal is hit by a car, or the family is away from home and a neighbour calls. Cattle, horses, and wild animals are found injured on the highway. Wildlife are found in traps or gunshot. Sick or starving pups and kittens are found in an alley. Pets are dumped by irresponsible owners. We veterinarians are constantly presented with patients for which there is no known owner. We treat these animals, and sometimes somebody comes forth to pay for the treatment and sometimes there is no owner or none can be found. Sometimes the owner is located but refuses to pay for the treatment, and we have no recourse in such cases because the owner is not obligated to pay for unauthorized services.

Most veterinarians come to accept this burden as a part of their career and become philosophical about it. Nearly all veterinarians find themselves rendering treatment free of charge to some livestock, pets, or wildlife.

So my statement to Mr Hayes was a bluff. I wanted him to feel bad.

I crossed the street and got into my car. 'Doctor!' a voice called out. Hayes came up to my window.

'I don't want to be responsible for that decision,' he said, taking out his cheque book. He wrote out a cheque for the full amount owed and handed it to me.

'If you had done this from the start, neither of us would have had to give up a half a day to be here,' I said.

'I'm a man of principle,' he answered. 'It was a matter of principle that made me refuse to pay the bill in the first place. After what you said, it's become a matter of principle that I pay it.'

'What if I told you that I was bluffing?' I asked. 'Suppose I just said it to make you feel guilty?'

'Perhaps you did, this time, but I'd be afraid that eventually you would make that decision, and I don't want it to be my fault,' he said. 'You know, I was just standing on my rights, and until you said that, I didn't realize that things like this must happen to you all the time. It's just once for me, but does this happen often for you?'

'Yes,' I responded, 'all the time. Today some people brought in a hawk with a broken wing and a sick kitten they found in an empty lot. We treated them, but there's nobody to bill. The hawk will be released, and we'll find someone to adopt the kitten. The only payment we receive is the satis-faction we get. That's why I took this to court, Mister

Hayes. There *is* an owner, and he *is* able to pay.'

'You're a decent man, Doctor Miller,' he said and extended his hand. I took it and told him, 'So are you, Mister Hayes.'

Chapter 25

'Teresa is only thirteen, but she knows that she wants to be a veterinarian,' said Mrs Klutterman. 'It's so kind of you to allow her to watch some surgery. Teresa, you watch quietly and don't bother the doctors. I'm going shopping and will be back to pick you up this afternoon.'

'Okay mom,' said Teresa, a solemn, quiet girl.

As I left the room to see patients up front, I heard Dr Kind say, 'Well, Teresa, the first thing we have to do is spay this little dog here. That's a panhysterectomy – removal of the uterus and the ovaries so Cindy won't have any unwanted puppies.'

Several minutes later Mary urgently approached me in the pharmacy.

'Dr Miller, Teresa fainted, and we think she hit her head on the concrete floor. You'd better go see.'

I hurried to the operating room where I found a distraught Bob Kind kneeling over the unconscious girl.

'I started an IV anaesthetic on the pup,' Bob said, 'and no sooner had I hit the vein when Teresa crashed down. Do you know where her mother went?'

'No,' I answered. 'Shopping somewhere, and she won't be back for several hours – look, she's regaining consciousness.'

Our community had grown to the point where half a dozen physicians had established practices, but several years were to elapse before we had a hospital. Of course, there was no ambulance service.

Teresa was conscious now and could communicate, but was showing definite signs of brain concussion. We had moved her to a comfortable bench and put a cushion under her head.

'Do you know where your mother is?' Mary asked.

'No.'

'Do you have a family doctor in town?'

'Yes.'

'What's his name?'

'I don't know, but he's young and good looking, and he is down the street.'

I quickly thought of the physicians in town and blurted out, 'Roy Larson!' Dr Larson seemed to fit the description.

'I have a patient under anaesthesia,' Bob said. 'Can you take her to the doctor?'

'Sure,' I replied. 'Mary, tell the people with appointments what happened, and I'll get back as soon as possible.'

Teresa was helped into my car; and still wearing my white office smock and stethoscope, I drove the girl to Roy Larson's office.

'I don't know her,' said Dr Larson. 'She's not my patient. I suggest that you leave her here, and we'll keep an eye on her.' I later learned that Dr James McGillis was the family doctor. Thousand Oaks was being enriched by the presence of young, handsome physicians. 'When Teresa's mother returns to your office, just send her here.'

I left the examining room and hurried down the hall towards the exit. As I passed the reception desk I saw Mrs McCarthy standing there. The receptionist was saying to Mrs McCarthy, 'Which doctor did you wish to see?'

'It doesn't matter,' said Mrs McCarthy, as she turned her head to see me striding towards her, my white coat fluttering and stethoscope dangling.

She pointed at me. 'Except him! He treats my horses!

What are *you* doing here Doctor Miller?'

'Good morning Mrs McCarthy,' I said breezily, passing. 'I work here part-time!'

'But,' she called after me, 'you treat my dogs and my horses. You treat *animals*!'

That's right,' I called as I disappeared around the corner. 'Most of the time! Most of my patients are animals!'

Most of my patients may be animals, but like all veterinarians, I occasionally find myself treating people, sometimes by design, but more often unintentionally. I have never delivered a human baby, but a colleague of mine did one night when a panic-stricken husband screeched up to his house with his wife in the back seat of the automobile in the final stages of labour.

'It was routine,' claims my friend. 'Just like delivering a puppy. . .'

I was practising in Thousand Oaks before any medical doctors located there, and my little clinic was equipped with an X-ray machine. The first three physicians who set up practice in town after I did had me do some of their routine radiographs. I soon learned that a frightened three-year-old child is a more difficult patient than most animals, simply because we veterinarians promptly sedate our patients for X-rays if they don't hold still. You don't do that with a child.

Emergencies on holidays have a way of fixing themselves in a veterinarian's memory. I remember the Christmas Eve, years ago, when a local physician asked me to radiograph an elderly woman's wrist. She had just stepped off a Greyhound bus, after arriving in town to visit her daughter and son-in-law, when she was struck by a car. The son-in-law, a client of mine, forever told people how his mother-in-law had been hit by a car, 'so they took her to the vet.'

Although we are trained and licensed to treat only animals, people inevitably will seek advice from veterinarians. We are careful to refer such people to their own

151

physicians but many amusing stories can be told because of this situation. Frequently, the owner has a problem similar to the animal's and without permission will take the animal's medication.

DMSO stands for dimethyl sulfoxide. It is an industrial solvent that was discovered to have some interesting medical properties. It was approved for use in horses many years ago. Most experienced horsepeople know this and are quite familiar with DMSO. Orthopaedic injuries and ailments are frequent in people who work with horses, and some of them resort to ingenious ruses to obtain the high-quality medical-grade DMSO manufactured for equine use.

When applied to human skin, DMSO quickly penetrates into the body and can soon be tasted in the mouth. It has a distinctive flavour and odour, which is often described as garlic-like or oyster-like. Among other uses, DMSO when applied to painful joints and muscles has an anti-inflammatory effect, and it relieves pain and swelling. The drug has not yet been approved by the Federal Drug Administration for human use, but it remains sought after nonetheless.

'Listen, Doc,' the old cowboy said. 'You've got some of that DMSO?' He put his left hand on his right shoulder and winced as he rotated his upper arm.

'It's for my old buckskin gelding – you know, my old roping horse. His – aah – his shoulder has been bothering him, I'd like to try some DMSO.'

'Well,' I replied, 'I'm not sure it's going to help him, but at least it will do no harm. Let's have a look at him.'

'Oh, he's up north, Doc, but I'll be seeing him this weekend. This stuff can't hurt him, can it? I mean, I know about the bad breath, but what the hell! It can't do anything bad to him, can it?'

'Well,' I said briskly, 'it can shrink the testicles, but since he's a gelding it doesn't matter, does it?'

He stopped rotating his arm and stared at me. I maintained a deadpan expression. Finally he snorted,

'Well, maybe I ought to blister that shoulder again, before I try anything new.'

A man approached me at a public stable. He wore a farrier's apron and carried some horse-shoeing tools. He was bent slightly forward at the waist and walked with short steps, moving mainly from the knees down. When he turned, he didn't rotate his head. He simply turned his entire body, stiffly. A dog, a Queensland heeler, frisked along behind him, tail wagging furiously. It raced around him in circles, lowered the front part of its body, yelped joyously, and then leaped high into the air.

The blacksmith pointed to the dog. 'He hurt his back,' he said. 'Hurts like hell. Can I use some of that ODMO on him?'

'What's that?' I asked.

'ODMO? You know! That garlic-tasting stuff you use on horses.'

'HEY, DOC!' the man greeted me. 'Can I have some of that DDSO?'

'What for?'

'For my horse!'

'What's wrong with him?'

He pointed to his own neck. 'He hurt an ankle!'

'May I see him?' I asked.

Reluctantly, the man left and returned with a brown gelding.

'Trot him out,' I suggested.

The horse moved soundly.

'He isn't lame,' I said.

'Right!' he agreed. 'Is it OK to use DDSO on his ankles to *prevent* an injury?'

Even prescribing medications for animals can require a certain subtle diplomacy – not that a horse or a cow cares what it's getting, but often the owner does.

153

Federal law in the United States requires that prescriptions, human or animal, be labelled with the name of the medication being used. This wasn't always true. Prescriptions for people used to be identified with mysterious code numbers, and it was common practice for veterinarians to re-label drugs. Many veterinary preparations came with removable labels to make the re-labelling easier.

Generally I preferred to leave labels on the drugs I dispensed. However, there are some people for whom a little knowledge is a dangerous thing. Sam Dickerson was such a man. A rancher, he loved to quack. He treated his own animals with every conceivable medication, and invariably he used the drugs improperly. So when I decided to put his sick calves on a long-acting form of penicillin, I knew that Sam would be better off if he didn't know what I was prescribing. I removed the label from a vial of the antibiotic and added a drop of Neoprontosil, a scarlet red antibacterial compound. The normally white penicillin turned a lovely pink.

'What is this stuff, Doc?' Sam wanted to know.

'It's long-acting antibiotic.'

'What's it called?'

'I mix it myself. I call it Erythromillercin.'

'Something new, huh?' said Sam. 'Looks like good stuff.'

I left instructions for the calves to be injected every other day. I knew that penicillin was the drug of choice for the sick animals, but penicillin is an innocent white in colour and available to stockmen at any feedstore or pharmacy selling veterinary drugs. If Sam didn't know what he was using and was impressed by the pink colour, the calves would be treated as I wanted them to be.

Sam came into the office a few days later. I asked how the calves were doing.

'They're all fine, Doc. The sick ones all got well, but now I got more sick and I'm outta that medicine you give me. I need more.'

I went into the pharmacy, removed the label from another vial of benzathine penicillin, added a drop of

Neoprontosil, and Sam happily went home to treat his cattle.

Two days later he was back in the office. 'Doc,' he said, 'I don't think the second vial of Erythromillercin was the same as the first.'

'Why not?' I asked.

'Well,' he said. 'First of all the second vial didn't work as good as the first. Them calves is still sick. In the second place, the first vial was pinker than the second.'

The colour of medication has a great psychological effect upon the person who uses it. I have noticed, with amusement, in a medical catalogue for humans, that aspirin tablets are available in six different colours, including green and red. Green and red are especially potent colours, even in a placebo. Every experienced practitioner is aware of the effect that the colour of a medication has upon the layman.

One of my veterinary school classmates, Dr Max Taylor, practised in Showlow, Arizona. One day Max was asked to geld a colt on the White River Apache Reservation. He put his instruments into a bucket of Nolvasan solution. Nolvasan is a bright blue disinfectant. Then to cast the colt, he injected succinylcholine intravenously. The colt collapsed, and a murmur went through the crowd of watching Indians.

Max finished the operation, and the colt soon staggered to its feet. Then the owner of the colt came forward, peered into the bucket of blue Nolvasan solution, and said, 'Boy! that's sure strong stuff!'

During an epidemic of equine influenza I was using a lot of intravenous erythromycin, a potent antibiotic that was new at the time. The Alabama-reared foreman of a Standardbred horse ranch watched me administer the clear, colourless solution. Somewhat apologetically, I said 'Looks like plain water, doesn't it?'

'Yeah, Doc,' he agreed. 'But I've seen a lot of good likker that colour.'

155

Chapter 26

Darlene Abbott was one of those people who make life difficult for veterinarians. She was a dog breeder with a kennel full of valuable show dogs. In addition, she owned several cats and three horses. She was well-off financially, having inherited some money, and was also probably receiving alimony from the most recent of her husbands. Darlene paid her bills reasonably well most of the time, was a dedicated fan of mine, sent me many new clients, and for these reasons ought to have been considered a valuable client. The problem with Darlene was that she was inconsiderate, self-centred, and demanding. She took an inordinate amount of my time during visits and over the telephone. She would speak to no one at the office but me, which did not serve to make her popular with Mary or Bob Kind. If I was unavailable, she saw my associate grudgingly, always managing to demean him in the process. Darlene demanded from me, and I'm afraid was accorded, a lot of time and attention. She managed to get my home telephone, which was unlisted, and called me at all hours, whether or not I was on call, to discuss problems with her animals. An intelligent woman, her animals' problems were never imagined, but real. In fact, she was a remarkably keen observer, and I learned to trust her judgment. When Darlene said an animal was 'not right,' I learned that her observation was invariably correct.

Darlene had great respect for my professional ability and vociferously praised me publicly among her many contacts in the animal world. I was not flattered by this, but I realized that it was an asset to our practice, and therefore, tolerated her many demands. When she exceeded the bounds of decency, however, I learned that I could bring her back into line by reprimanding her and firmly saying, 'No!' For example, she liked to feel that she owned the hospital, striding into the operating room or wards uninvited, sitting beside one of her hospitalized animals for hours on end, and upsetting the staff by barking orders to my assistant or loudly calling to me, 'Bob, I think her temperature is going up again. Bob, better come back here and check her.' As I said, she was usually correct. She was not a hypochondriac. However, it was difficult to work and think under such conditions, in which case I would say, 'Darlene, you are upsetting our routine and interfering with our ability to take care of our many patients. Please go home.' Whereupon, with a contrite expression, she would obediently go home like a chastised little girl, only to telephone an hour later, wanting immediate and lengthy reports, from me personally, as to the patient's condition.

I am tolerant of people's idiosyncrasies, always trying to interpret why they behave as they do, and since Darlene was a sincere animal lover, her concern extended to animals other than those she personally owned. Our relationship went on for many years, until she finally moved elsewhere.

Once I had a bad cold. In those days, I would 'work away' a cold. In fact, several times I had gone skiing with a cold and come home well. I didn't believe in pampering myself. By the end of the week in question, however, I looked forward to my Sunday off and decided to spend it in bed. After working all week with a nagging respiratory infection, I hoped that a day's rest would revive me while Bob Kind took care of the emergencies. I had fallen asleep over a book when Debby woke me up. 'Darlene Abbott is at the door. She needs to speak to you right away. I told her you were sick.' Darlene lived in our neighbourhood.

With conflicting emotions, I went to the door. 'Oh, Bob,' she said, 'I'm so glad you're home. A group of people were riding their horses down in the barranca right behind your house, and one of the horses is stuck in quicksand.'

It was January, California's rainy season, and it was a wet winter. Behind my home was a stream, in a gully about forty feet deep which we called by its Spanish name, the barranca. The stream, greatly swollen by the rains, would develop areas of quicksand, and one of these areas was directly behind and below our house.

'Her head is all that is showing out of the quicksand, and they found a piece of plywood to put under it, but she is slowly sinking.' I quickly put on my clothes and a pair of knee-high rubber boots, grabbed some ropes from the barn, and slid and grappled my way down the steep barranca wall to the stream. There, just as Darlene had described, were a bunch of frantic riders, all but one of their horses tied to trees. That one, a palomino mare, was lying on her side, only her head, neck, and one shoulder were visible, supported by a sheet of plywood. Her saddle and bridle had been removed and she wore a halter. Four youngsters were futilely pulling on the halter rope.

'We've sent for the fire department and rescue squad,' somebody said.

'Then we've got to pass a rope around her body, behind her forelegs,' I replied. 'You can't get her out of there by the neck.'

Even as I spoke, I could see the mare, who was too tired to struggle, sinking deeper into the swirling bottomless sand. Her head was closest to the bank and a volunteer slid down, wedging his leg under the plywood to help keep the mare's nose above water. Meanwhile I waded in to pass a rope around the mare's middle. In seconds the icy water flowed over my boot tops. It was the first and only time in my life that I've ever been in quicksand. As I struggled to pass the rope under the mare, the quicksand insidiously sucked me down until I was waist deep. The lower half of my body was immovable and numb with cold. I wasn't worried because there were many people on the bank with ropes to pull me out if I sank too far in. After a half-hour's unsuccessful attempts to work a rope under the mare, a fire department rescue truck and bulldozer showed up on the opposite bank. The dozer worked its way down to the stream, and a fireman on the opposite side of the mare was able to reach the rope I passed to him under her body. I had been in the cold water for over an hour before the dozer was able to pull the mare out of the quicksand onto solid ground. I went home, got my practice truck, and drove it to the closest bridge and made my way cross-country to the mare. She was now on the opposite bank, and this necessitated a two-mile drive. I found her still down, paralysed with fatigue and hypothermia, and I sincerely doubted if she would ever get up. While volunteers rubbed her dry, I catheterized a vein and, to stimulate the mare and help her fight shock, loaded her with glucose solution, amphetamine, and a massive dose of cortisone derivative. Thus fortified, she struggled to her feet after I goaded her with an electric cattle prod. We all cheered. After a final injection of penicillin to ward off infection in her weakened state, the mare was led home. She recuperated uneventfully. However, I developed pneumonia afterwards, took weeks to recuperate, and I have had trouble shaking off a cold ever since. I don't catch colds very often, but when I do, they nearly always terminate with a persistent bronchial cough.

Sometimes difficult clients drive their friendly veterinarian to engage in little games of vengeance.

One of our clients, whom I'll call Merv Pill, is extremely demanding. He used to insist on precise times for appointments and go into a tantrum if we were late. Keeping exact appointments is difficult in large-animal practice because we never know how much time each visit will require, and our routine is frequently interrupted by emergencies.

We can usually tell clients what day we'll arrive, and often we can tell them whether it will be in the morning or afternoon, but rarely can we commit ourselves to an exact hour. To placate Merv, my partner told him that he would deworm and vaccinate his herd at exactly 8:30 a.m. on a Saturday morning in February and that he would confirm the appointment at 8 a.m.

It poured rain the entire day before Merv's appointment and was still raining on Saturday morning. Bob knew that the farm would be a mire and that everything would be cold and miserable as he telephoned Merv at 8 a.m.

'Good morning!' he said cheerily, 'I'm on my way!'

'But,' Merv protested, 'the rain's coming down in sheets.'

'No problem,' said Bob, clad in boots and slicker. 'I'll be there at eight-thirty, just as I promised!'

Merv never again demanded an exact time for an appointment.

Another client – we'll call her Gladys Bubbly – woke me one midnight in March.

'My mare is foaling,' she babbled. 'Something's wrong! She's taking too long!'

'Go back and look at her again!' I said, using my technique for uncertain dystocia calls. 'I'll hold the phone and get ready to leave.'

Most such calls are false alarms. If the caller returns to the phone in a minute to say there is no change, I leave immediately. But, few clients get back to the phone in less than five minutes. When this happens, I know that the foal has emerged and the caller is so busy admiring it that he or she has forgotten about me.

About ten minutes went by, and I was dozing off with the telephone cradled to my ear when Mrs Bubbly came back on the line.

'Doctor? Oh, I'm sorry I kept you so long. Everything is fine. We have a beautiful filly!'

'Congratulations,' I said. 'I'll be by first thing in the morning to do the postpartum examination. Save the placenta for me to see.'

I was asleep when the phone rang at 1 a.m. It was Mrs Bubbly.

'Doctor, there's something wrong with the foal. It's uncoordinated. It struggles to its feet, but is very wobbly and falls down.'

'That's rather normal for an hour-old foal,' I explained patiently. Mrs Bubbly should have known better because she had observed at least a dozen foalings.

Half an hour later, just as I was falling asleep, the phone rang again. 'Is it normal for the foal to cough and sputter and have fluids running out of its nose?'

'Is it up and around now?' I asked.

'Yes, and it seems stronger. It's a big foal.'

'Sounds normal,' I said. 'There is usually some mucus and placental fluid in the respiratory tract, and it takes a while for those to be expelled or absorbed.'

I slept for two and half hours before the phone rang again. It was 4 a.m.

'Doctor,' said Mrs Bubbly. 'Something is wrong with this foal. It starts to nurse, then seems to lose the teat. It noses around for a while before finding the teat again.'

'Does it nurse strongly?' I asked.

'Oh, yes! It seems very greedy.'

'Sounds quite normal for a foal just beginning to nurse,' I said wearily. 'You haven't told me anything that concerns me. I'll see the mare and foal in the morning.'

I awoke at 5:30 a.m., as I always do, despite interruptions. At 6 a.m., I went to the telephone in the kitchen so as not to waken the rest of the family. I dialled Mrs Bubbly's home. The phone rang several times before a garbled voice answered.

'Hello?'

'Good morning,' I boomed enthusiastically. 'This is Doctor Miller. How is our foal this morning?'

'Don't know,' the voice mumbled sleepily. 'Went to sleep an hour ago. Don't know.'

'Well,' I sparkled, 'I'll be at your place in thirty minutes. Meet me at the barn.'

When I arrived, Mrs Bubbly was there, face puffed and eyes squinting with fatigue. Before leaving, I noted that the foal's right flexor tendon was slightly contracted. I directed Mrs Bubbly to spend the next two hours gently extending the fetlock to stretch the tendon. I left her hunched over the foal, whimpering softly in the morning fog.

I drove home for breakfast filled with satisfaction. It was going to be a good day. Mrs Bubbly had a fine new foal, and I felt sure that she would never again phone asking me to see a healthy, normal foal until after the sun was up.

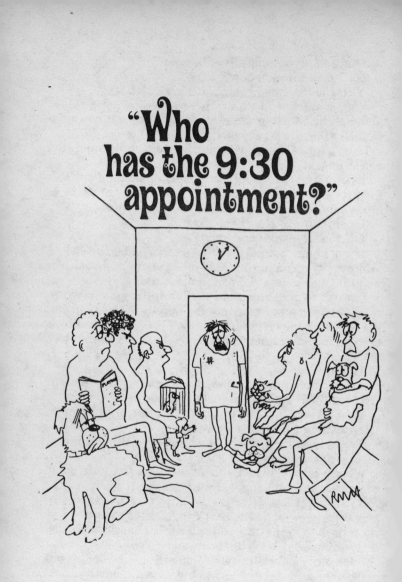

162

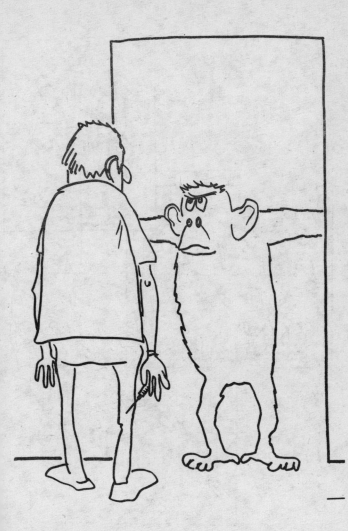

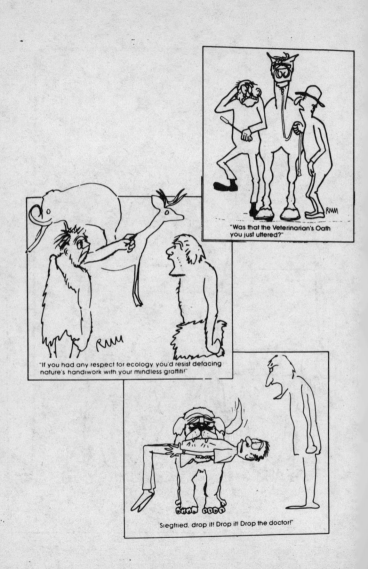

"Was that the Veterinarian's Oath you just uttered?"

"If you had any respect for ecology, you'd resist defacing nature's handiwork with your mindless graffiti!"

"Siegfried, drop it! Drop it! Drop the doctor!"

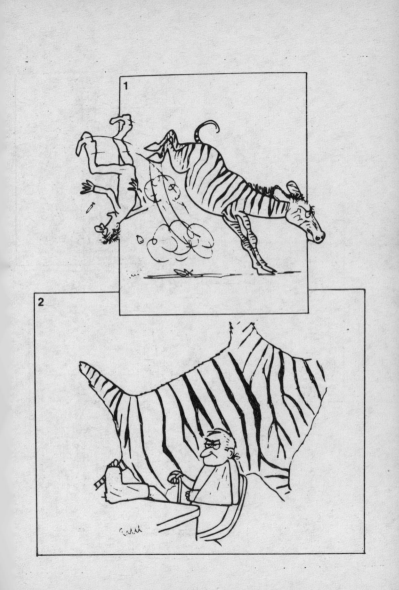

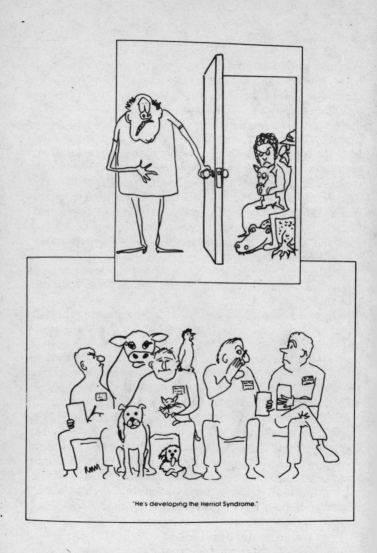

"He's developing the Herriot Syndrome."

Chapter 27

As soon as I heard the automobile screeching to a stop in front of our clinic door, I knew that an emergency was coming in. Mary and I were talking about some business problems at her desk. We turned to look out the window. A distraught woman rushed out of the car, holding a limp puppy in her arms. I opened the door for her. She stopped in front of me. Her face was ashen, her eyes wide with terror, and she was trembling uncontrollably. She could not speak, but quavering agonizing sounds came from her lips. Taking the pup from her, I quickly moved it to an examination table. The puppy was alive, but unconscious, and I knew at once that its injuries were fatal. As I checked the grey mucous membranes and listened to its labouring chest, I asked, 'Run over?'

She nodded, still unable to speak and still making those incoherent whimpering sounds. Her hands fluttered uncontrollably.

'I'll try,' I said, and picked up the limp mongrel puppy and disappeared through the door leading to the treatment room. Sticking the pup's muzzle into an oxygen mask, I turned on the NCG resuscitator and then grabbed an intravenous cut-down pack and a bottle of gelatin plasma substitute, hoping that an intravenous injection of plasma would somehow reverse what I knew was fatal shock.

With an electric clipper I quickly shaved a forearm, put a tourniquet on the leg, but then I stopped. I was too late. The puppy had died. The heart beat was gone. I felt the warm soft belly. It was distended with internal haemorrhage. For a moment I stood there, realizing that I had to go back into the examining room to tell the shocked woman what had happened. I shut off the resuscitator and slowly walked to the door.

'Is he your own puppy?' I asked.

She nodded. Still unable to speak, she continued to

167

shudder and kept making those awful whimpering sounds.

'Did you run over him yourself?' Her reaction had been so extreme in what was, unfortunately, a rather common emergency situation, that I had inferred that she herself had injured the pup rather than somebody else.

Now she spoke for the first time.

'I backed over him. He was in the driveway and I backed over him.' It was hoarsely whispered.

'Why don't you sit down?' I suggested. She was in such an extreme state that I was afraid of what might happen when I announced the puppy's death.

Mary came into the room, a concerned and sympathetic look on her face. She led the woman to a chair, then left us together, softly closing the door behind her.

'Will he be all right?' the woman asked. Her teeth chattered as she spoke, and her voice was choked.

'I'm sorry, but he's gone.'

Her eyes rolled up in her head, and she let out a wail that made my skin crawl. Then she began to cry and sob hysterically and uncontrollably.

'Must be emotionally unstable,' I thought to myself. Her grief was so extreme, her reaction so severe that I realized that there was more wrong here than just the loss of a puppy. She was inconsolable.

Eventually the woman told us who she was, and when I suggested that she not drive home by herself, she gave us a neighbour's telephone number to call.

The neighbour quickly came to the clinic and, showing great concern, led the shattered woman to her car. She then came back into the office and told us that the crying woman's husband would come in later in the day to pick up his wife's car and to take care of any charges.

'Is she all right?' I asked. 'I can understand her grief and her feelings of guilt, but her reaction is so extreme. I've never seen anybody react that way, especially over the death of a puppy. It was only a few months of age. People usually don't become that deeply attached to a dog unless they have owned it for many years.'

The neighbour, a kindly middle-aged person, looked at me and tears welled into her eyes. And then she explained.

'One day she killed both of her own children the same way – backed over them in the driveway.'

The horror of that story overwhelmed me and has never left me. After I had children of my own, I often stopped abruptly while backing out of the driveway and got out of the car with a sense of apprehension and checked to be sure there were no toddlers behind me. Even today, a quarter of a century after the incident, I check for children and dogs before backing up. I drive more than a hundred miles on an average working day, making my rounds, and I constantly have to back out of driveways to barns and stables. All of the vehicles I drive are fitted with oversize rear-view side mirrors. The tragedies of that woman's life are seared into my memory.

Chapter 28

Wild-animal trainers are a special breed of people – especially those who train the big cats.

George Keller was a college professor, the head of the department of visual arts and dean of men at the State Teacher's College at Bloomsburg, Pennsylvania. Professor Keller had always loved animals.

From boyhood, he had a secret dream of being a lion tamer, starring in the centre ring of *The Greatest Show on Earth*. His schoolmates had often been amused by his efforts to train dogs, cats, and other domestic animals.

Years later, after he had become a respected college faculty member, a former fraternity brother sent him a live, full grown mountain lion as a joke. Attached to the cage was a note, which said: 'Here Keller – train this.'

The professor did exactly that. He trained the mountain lion in his backyard. Over time he bought several big cats and soon had an impressive act going in a cage on his property. At first he did benefit performances with his cats, but eventually an agent saw him and offered him a summer's booking in Atlantic City, New Jersey. George Keller, college professor, became a professional lion tamer.

After a couple of seasons, he realized that he was experiencing more joy in life as a performer than he did as a teacher. George Keller felt that middle age needn't be a barrier to a complete change in one's way of life or to a drastic change in occupation. He believed that one can accomplish one's dream if one has determination and conviction. Past fifty years of age, Keller left his teaching and administrative position and went on the road with an act of mixed big cats. Lions, tigers, leopards, jaguar, and puma all performed together in the circus ring in an exciting and action-filled act. For years Keller struggled to reach the top, enduring the uncertainties and the hardships of circus life. He was aided in his perseverance by his wife, Virginia, who years later would come to work at the Conejo Valley Veterinary Clinic.

There were long intervals without bookings. During these times there were often financial hardships. Lions and tigers must eat regularly. There were frightening moments, as when the animals were poisoned, an incident mentioned earlier. When Keller and company weren't on the road, they resided on their ranch a few miles from Thousand Oaks, practising their act every day in a big circus-style round cage. Their neighbours grew used to the roaring and the sound of cracking whips and blank pistol shots used during the act. When bookings were available, it meant strenuous travel across the country, living the nomadic gypsy life of circus folks.

After nine years of this existence, a man called upon them at the ranch that served as their winter quarters and training centre. He was an agent for the Ringling Brothers Barnum and Bailey Circus. Keller's Jungle Killers, as the act was known, made the centre ring. George Keller's boyhood dream of being a lion tamer in *The Greatest Show on Earth* had become reality.

Keller wrote a book, a fascinating autobiography called *Here Keller, Train This*. Those were the words written on the note attached to the cage with the mountain lion that Keller's friend had sent as a prank.

George Keller died at sixty-one years of age. He went with his boots on, suffering a heart attack in the middle of his act, surrounded by the great cats he loved.

Dick Walker also had a boyhood dream of becoming a lion tamer. As a young man he went to Jungleland and offered to work for nothing, just to be near the big cats and the trainers he envied and admired. He learned the trade the hard way, starting out by cleaning cages and doing chores. By the time Debby and I had moved to Thousand Oaks, Dick had reached the top of his field. He had an impressive act, using nothing but huge male lions. His act was world famous and was featured in circuses, television productions, and motion pictures. I saw Dick in a television show called *Danger Is My Business*. While being interviewed on that show, he explained that the fascination in his chosen career was two-fold. First of all, there was the love he had for his majestic and powerful beasts. Second, he was enamoured of the danger in his business. The risk and the excitement were what made life interesting for him. An extremely intelligent, articulate, serious man, Dick was always a pleasure to speak with. His was a profession that only a handful of people in the entire world had mastered, and I greatly enjoyed knowing people like him and having them as clients.

I had known Dick Walker for several years when I ran

into him one day at a local food market. I hadn't seen him in quite a while.

'Hello, Dick,' I said. 'How are the cats?'

He looked surprised. 'Why, haven't you heard? I quit the animal business!'

'Really?' I replied. 'What are you doing now?'

'Doc, when a man reaches the age of forty and is tied to a routine job and doesn't have his heart in it, and all the time there's something he wants to do more than anything else in the world – he's got to make the change then or he probably never will.'

'So,' I asked, 'what are you doing now?'

'I mean,' he continued, 'it was the same routine day after day; down to the park, work the act, crack the whip, mess with the lions, with only occasional bookings to relieve the monotony, and all the time I'm burning to do something new.'

'Like what?' I asked, 'what are you doing now?'

'It wasn't *easy* to make this change. I had a successful act, and it took me a long time to reach that point. I have a family to support. The *easy* thing to do would have been to keep on with it, stay in the rut, and put my personal ambitions aside. I mean, I've had to start all over. I had to train for a new career at the mid-point in my life. But I knew that if I didn't have the guts to start over and do what I really wanted to do, I'd probably never do it if I didn't do it now – and so I did it!'

'Did what?' I was now consumed with curiosity.

'And I'm *happy*! I'm doing what I wanted to. I'm glad I did it!'

'Dick,' I implored, 'what are you doing?'

'I'm operating a computer.'

Chapter 29

The role of house pets as surrogate children is well recognized within the veterinary profession. When extremely close bonding occurs between a human and an animal, the most frequent role the pet is playing is as a substitute child. There is nothing abnormal in this relationship. Indeed, it verifies the strong instinct in our own species to live in family groups. Dogs especially, being themselves members of a species that lives in packs, fit the surrogate role admirably, thus explaining the ancient symbiotic relationship between humans and canines. Prehistoric man kept dogs, and they hunted together, fought together, protected one another, and each warded off the other's loneliness. The fact that man has often abused the dog, and even used him for food, does not alter the depth or the importance of the relationship between the two species. Man has often abused and even eaten his own species, yet he always needed other humans to live with and for.

In 1961 Thousand Oaks was still a country village. Bob Kind and I attended a meeting of the San Fernando Valley Veterinary Association. Unlike the Conejo Valley, the San Fernando Valley was a suburban extension of huge and sprawling Los Angeles. San Fernando's monthly veterinary meeting gave my partner and myself an opportunity to listen to good speakers and learn of scientific advances in our profession.

Over dinner the talk, as always, was about our patients, their diseases, and their owners. One of our big-city colleagues made an interesting comment. He observed that homosexual couples were often the most dedicated of pet owners because, he thought, unlike heterosexual couples, the pet represented the only possible 'children' they could have. (This was before homosexual couples started adopting children.) There was immediate and affirmative agreement from most of the men at the table. (This was also before women veterinarians became commonplace, so all of the veterinarians present were men.)

Bob and I looked at each other uncomprehendingly. There were no obviously homosexual couples bringing pets to our office.

'Is this common?' I asked. 'Do you have a lot of homosexual clients coming in with pets as part of the family?'

The veterinarians present assured us that this was a common phenomenon, indeed, and within a few years, as our town grew and became a commuting community, several such couples joined our clientele. They were, as we had been told, intensely devoted to their pets. I noticed that in most cases, they selected a pet of the same sex as their own. Male homosexuals living together nearly always had a male pet, and the females had a female.

Two nurses who lived together had a miniature schnauzer named Heidi whom they loved dearly and took extraordinarily good care of. The women made no effort to conceal their lesbian relationship. They were ideal clients for a veterinarian, being considerate and appreciative, and since they were registered nurses, they understood the technical aspects of their dog's illnesses better than most lay people.

One day they brought Heidi in. The dog was in terrible pain. After examining her, I told the owners that I suspected an attack of acute pancreatitis, and I ran some laboratory tests which soon confirmed the diagnosis. Although I had treated Heidi for a variety of minor ailments before, she had never required hospitalization. This time, however, she was very sick.

'I'll need to keep her and hook her up to an IV,' I said.

'Oh no, Doctor Miller,' they protested. 'We can't leave her. Tell us what to do, and we'll do it. We're nurses, and we can give her injections or whatever she needs.'

'Look,' I said. 'I've never asked you to leave her here before because she has never been this sick. She is desperately ill, needs intensive care, and I can't do what's best for her unless you leave her with me.'

Both women had tears in their eyes. 'Doctor,' said one of them, 'this is not just a dog to us. She is our child. We can't leave her.'

'I know that, and I understand,' I assured her. 'I know what she means to you, and that's exactly why you must leave her. I want to save her for you, and I can't if you don't hospitalize her.'

The other woman said, 'But you don't understand. *She is our child. I mean this literally!*'

'I *do* understand!' I said, looking at both of them and my expression must have told them that I did. 'I *understand*. I *know* what she means to you, and I'm going to do all that I can to save her.'

Heidi spent several days at our clinic. She was near death at one point. Bob and I took turns taking her home at night, keeping her in a small cage near our bed, and Heidi got well. When we returned her to her tearful and happy owners, two women who would never know natural motherhood but who were nevertheless filled with maternal love and longing, Heidi weakly but happily wagged her tail. She was glad to be going home.

I also recall two women who came all the way from Hollywood with their one-year-old pet chimpanzee. They called the little chimp Tricia and had it dressed in expensive pink baby clothes.

'She has a bad leg,' one of them explained.

After I removed the little animal's pink panties and diapers, I said, 'She's a boy!'

'Yes, we know, but we wanted a girl chimp, and this was the only one we could find, so we just pretend it's a girl.' (They always insisted on referring to the chimp as 'she'.)

The chimp had a deformed knee. After I X-rayed it, the reason was obvious. There were two buck-shot pellets in the small ape's body. One was in its back and the other near one shoulder. It was common to find buck shot in pet shop primates. No doubt a native hunter had shot the mother chimpanzee out of the trees. The baby clinging to her back

175

had been wounded and probably had injured its knee during the fall. The native had then sold the baby to a wild-animal dealer, and eventually the chimp had reached a pet shop in California.

This animal was fortunate. It had survived long enough to be placed in a private home and was being fed well, even though it had to endure diapers and frilly, pink dresses. Most animals captured in this way died of disease or malnutrition long before they reached an American pet shop.

Now the chimp's right patella had disintegrated, probably the result of that neglected fracture which occurred during the fall from the trees in far-off Africa.

I looked at the owners. One of them was a beautiful young woman. She was a singer, and I later saw her on television. She was feminine, stylishly dressed, sexy, and as I said, beautiful. Her eyes were grey, her hair long and blond. As I spoke, she responded with animated conversation and a warm smile.

The other woman was different. She was a big woman, dressed in sloppy jeans and a blue, man's work shirt. Her face was plain and mannish, her black hair cut extremely short, almost in a crew cut, and her fingernails were short and grimy.

As I discussed the case, I became aware of the hostility of this second woman. I was puzzled why she met every statement I made with a snide or derisive comment.

Increasingly, I directed my remarks to the pretty, pleasant owner. This seemed to antagonize her companion even more. Then I realized what I was doing wrong. I wasn't acknowledging the head of the family.

As soon as I understood why I had lost rapport with one half of the family, I diplomatically altered my tactics. I stopped looking at the beautiful owner and maintained eye contact with the other one. Immediately, I could see a change in her demeanour. From then on, I made all my suggestions to 'Dad,' while 'Mom' cuddled and crooned to little Tricia, and soon we all understood each's relationship to the other three. I was the paediatrician and Dad was definitely the head of the family. Dad paid the bills and made the decisions – and made sure that nobody messed with the little woman.

I consulted with an orthopaedic surgeon on this case. Today we have board certified veterinary orthopaedists, but there were none in those days so I used an MD Actually, the chimp's knee was identical with a human baby's knee, anyway. In fact, Dr Les Cohn asked if he could take the X-ray films to show to his colleagues of UCLA, and none of them was aware that the patient wasn't human.

Dr Cohn kindly offered to operate on the knee at no charge, and the little chimp had a functional knee post-surgically.

Probably the clearest indication that pets often serve as surrogate children is the way their owners refer to them. For example, what are clients likely to say when they realize the drug prescribed for their pet is also used by human beings? Do they say, 'Oh, this is the same thing that people take?' No, they usually say, 'Oh, that's the same thing grownups take.' Or 'Does Fido take it the same way an adult does?'

Many clients are dismayed to hear a veterinarian refer to their pet as an animal. Some owners don't even like their pets called dogs or cats. The tactful practitioner soon learns to call patients by name.

'Prince has a bladder stone,' is more acceptable to owners than, 'Your animal has a bladder stone.' Veterinarians should remember that Prince is a member of the family.

Veterinarians who regularly treat zoo animals kept as pets see some unusual relationships between these animals and their owners. In a practice where exotic animals are treated, one can expect anything.

In my early years in practice, I discovered an effective treatment for simian bone disease. This fatal disease was, at that time, the most common cause of death in pet monkeys. It was also known as cage paralysis and was often thought to be caused by lack of exercise.

Eventually, the disease was correctly identified as nutritional secondary hyperparathyroidism. Pet monkeys were usually fed only fruits and nuts. This calcium-deficient diet caused irreversible metabolic abnormalities and skeletal deformities. Dozens of pet monkeys with grotesquely contorted limbs and skulls were brought to our clinic for treatment. The disease is rarely seen today because balanced commercial diets are available for primates.

Harry and Dolly Carter came to our clinic with three woolly monkeys that were suffering from simian bone disease. Harry, a man in his mid-sixties, owned a burlesque theatre in Los Angeles. His wife, Dolly, was more than thirty-five years his junior. She was a stripper and danced in Harry's theatre. Our practice was a long drive from downtown LA, but Harry and Dolly didn't mind because they were so pleased to find veterinarians who were willing to treat their pets and who knew about the diseases of monkeys.

The Carters came to see us regularly. As the condition of their monkeys improved, their delight was obvious. The monkeys, which were less enthusiastic about the visits, came dressed in little suits that Dolly had made. For the Carters, the business of burlesque was only a way to make money. What really mattered to them was their monkeys. Children could not have had more parental love lavished on them than did those monkeys.

One day, after the Carters left the office, I said to my partner, 'Bob, isn't it tragic that people cannot recognize their needs? There goes a couple aching for children. They need a real family. Why don't they adopt a couple of orphans and give them the time, money, and love they give those monkeys?'

The Carters were good clients. They followed instructions, were appreciative of our efforts, paid their bills promptly, and did not take up an unreasonable amount of our time. Granted, they came into our office bearing monkeys dressed like children, but they could not be classified as crackpots. They simply suffered from an overdose of parental longing, and the monkeys served as surrogate children. I kept hoping the Carters would recognize their need and adopt a child.

Several years passed. One day the Carters came in with a monkey. With them they brought a little girl. Bonnie, a neatly dressed four-year-old, was pretty and bright. While Mary entertained Bonnie, Dolly and Harry told me of the little girl's plight.

'Bonnie's mother was one of our strippers. She wasn't married, and she was a heroin addict. She neglected that precious child and then ran off to Europe with some bum and told us to take care of Bonnie.'

The Carters' faces gleamed with enthusiasm as they told me what a wonderful child Bonnie was. They were malevolent when they spoke of her mother. 'How could a woman – any woman – abandon her own flesh and blood?' Dolly asked. 'And what a child! How could her mother leave her?'

Harry said, 'We're going to keep her! We're going to adopt Bonnie and give her a good home.'

I was so pleased. Even if it meant the loss of the monkey business, I was happy for the Carters and for little Bonnie. Fate had intervened. A couple who needed a child had found a child who needed a home.

I did not see the Carters for several months. Then, one day, Dolly called. One of the monkeys had a skin lesion. It didn't sound serious, but I couldn't diagnose the problem without seeing it. She said she'd drive out in the morning.

When Dolly and Bonnie came in with the monkey Bonnie said, 'I want to watch.'

'Okay,' said Dolly impatiently, and holding the monkey in one arm, she led Bonnie into the examination room with her other hand. She put the monkey, wrapped in a soft receiving blanket, on the table.

She then turned to Bonnie, pointed to the bench, and

179

said sharply, 'Bonnie! Sit!' Bonnie climbed up on the bench and sat. Next, Dolly raised her hand, arm extended toward the little girl, and said, 'Bonnie! Stay!'

Dolly turned toward me, unwrapped the blanket, and started to tell me about the spot on the monkey's arm. But I couldn't concentrate on what she was saying because of the devastating scene I had just witnessed: a pet treated like a child and a child treated like a pet.

About a year later, Harry came in alone. He looked haggard. 'How is Mrs Carter?' I asked.

'She left me,' he said. 'Left me with the monkeys and Bonnie. Ran off with a twenty-five-year-old guy. I can't believe it! I can believe she'd leave me. I'm too damn old for her anyway. And I can believe she'd leave Bonnie. After all, she's not her own flesh and blood. But I can't believe she left the monkeys. I never thought she'd do that!'

The roles pets play in people's lives vary to extremes. A vivid example of one extreme came not from my practice, but from an incident I witnessed on a weekend I was off visiting a friend who lived in San Bernardino. Looking out of his kitchen window, I saw a large California box tortoise crawling about his back yard.

I asked, 'Dick, your yard isn't fenced. Why doesn't that tortoise wander off the property?'

'What tortoise?' Dick asked.

'That one!' I pointed at the lumbering reptile.

Dick looked out the window.

'That's not my tortoise,' he said, 'but I think I know where it came from.'

At the back of his property, thick shrubbery separated Dick's yard from a neighbour's. We poked our way through the shrubbery until we could look into the neighbour's yard. An old couple were gardening. Scattered about the yard we could see a half a dozen more tortoises.

'Have you lost a tortoise?' Dick called. The old people stood up looking in all directions and up in the air for the mysterious voice.

'Over here,' said Dick. 'In the shrubbery!'

Having located the source of the voice, they hurried over and accepted the tortoise my friend held out.

'It's Elmer, Mother!' said the old man.

'Elmer's come home!'

Without another word to us they both cuddled the tortoise and walked towards the house, covering it with kisses.

'Elmer,' the woman scolded. 'You bad boy! Where have you been? Your brothers and sisters and Mother and Daddy have been worried sick about you. It's been weeks, you bad boy! Where have you been?'

My friend, who was raised on an Idaho ranch, squinted at me and spat on the ground. 'You're a vet,' he said. 'You ever see anybody kiss a turtle before?'

A tale like this needs an opposite extreme for emphasis and contrast. So I'll tell you about Greg, a client of mine who is a commercial airline pilot. His daughter had a pet marc who was a 'member of the family.' One day he called and asked me to examine the mare for lameness. The old animal had ringbone, and the arthritis had advanced to a degree where little could be done and she was no longer safe to ride.

'Well,' he said, 'I couldn't sell her to anybody else with a clear conscience, and she's an old pet that the kids have loved, so I really can't put her through an auction and have some dog food company buy her. I guess there's really nothing to do but put her out of her misery.'

I reluctantly agreed with his decision. 'So,' he said, 'I guess we'll fatten her up, and in a month or so we'll ask you about destroying her.'

I was puzzled. 'Fatten her up?' I asked.

'Sure,' he said. 'She'll be better eating if we fatten her up, won't she? Like a steer?'

'Better eating?' I was still perplexed.

'Yes! Isn't that OK? I mean horsemeat is good to eat isn't it? They eat it in Europe. No sense wasting her. We'll fatten her up, and then we'll have her slaughtered and put the

181

meat in the locker.'

Despite the logic of his argument, I was relieved to learn that the rest of the family vetoed his plan. His wife and daughter had no intention of devouring the old horse which had been a friend and companion for so long.

As you know by now, mine is not an ordinary practice. I've had my share of distinctive patients, and Cookie ranks right up near the top. In fact, Cookie even sent me an invitation to his birthday party. He had recovered and was celebrating.

Cookie is a caiman, a South American crocodilian. He was only eight inches long when he came from the pet shop. When first presented to me by the owner, a Hungarian widow who talked like Zsa-Zsa Gabor and looked the way Zsa-Zsa might look without the benefits of modern cosmetology, Cookie had attained a length of five feet and weight of thirty-five pounds. Cookie had a blue ribbon tied around his neck, and his head was covered with lipstick stains. Accompanied by a friend who kept nodding agreement and murmuring. 'It's true – everything she says is true,' Cookie's owner told me about her pet's history and problems.

Cookie slept in a basket beside the owner's bed. I was told Cookie was afraid of water. Though timid, Cookie answered to his name. Cookie knew when Mother was going on a trip, because he would grow morose when he saw the suitcases being packed. He refused to eat unless he was told, 'Cookie is going on a trip! We won't leave Cookie at home this time!' Cookie had been around the world seven times with his owner and her husband, a scientist.

The reptile loved to ride in the back of an automobile, stretched out along the back window. Service station attendants, cleaning the rear window and assuming that Cookie was a stuffed specimen, often reeled back in horror when Cookie made a sudden move.

On one trip, a baggage porter seized Cookie from the lady and started to carry him away, along with an armload of suitcases. Shortly, luggage flew in all directions, accompanied by a shriek, 'It's alive!'

Cookie lived on a diet of hamburger, and therein lies the source of his ailment. The calcium-deficient diet had caused the same nutritional problems that used to afflict pet monkeys. Consequently his bones had softened. Cookie had back pain, and his teeth were giving him trouble.

'I vant you should examine his teeth, Doctor,' the owner said. Her friend nodded support.

Cookie was on the examining table. He trembled as I have seen so many dogs do, afraid of the doctor. I understood. I was afraid of the patient. I bent over to examine him, fillcd with professional interest, my hands clasped tightly behind my back.

'Vill you look at his teeth, Doctor?' the owner asked again.

'Ah? How – uh – how do we get his mouth open?' I responded. I could hear stifled giggles outside the examination room, where Mary and Bob had gathered to see how I handled this most exotic of exotic pets.

'Cookie!' the lady commented. 'Open your mouth for ze nice doctor!'

To my amazement, the creature's jaw grew slack, and I could easily examine the teeth. They were loose. Cookie's shaking became more violent as my confidence increased.

'Vait, Doctor!' the woman suggested. She bent over Cookie's head. 'Sveetheart!' she crooned. 'Doctor von't hurt you. Don't be afraid. Doctor is nice man.'

Cookie, unbelievably, stopped shaking, slowly relaxed and lowered his elevated forequarters down to the table, and sighed.

I spent three-quarters of an hour prescribing for Cookie and listening with growing fascination to his owner's tales. When I bid her goodbye, I confessed to her, 'You know, when you first began to tell me of your relationship with this reptile, I thought you were a crackpot. I see now that there is actual rapport between you. He understands you, and he responds to you. Frankly, I always assumed that a crocodile had the intelligence of a carrot, but you have opened my eyes. The level of communication you have with this animal is far higher than I thought possible. I learned something today.'

The woman's eyes sparkled. 'Doctor,' she said, 'nefer underestimate ze power of love!'

Chapter 30

I have always welcomed patients of all species, for the fun and challenge of it and because of the variety of exotic animals in southern California. As a result, I have encountered the gamut of unusual situations. (I once treated a whale and a hummingbird on the same day!)

Among the exotic cases that stand out in my memory are a lion that swallowed a cane, a kangaroo that collided head-on with a car on the highway, a sunburned whale, and a constipated elephant.

On one occasion, I sutured a laceration on a ten-foot boa constrictor that had crawled through a broken window. Two weeks later the owner brought the snake in a sack for removal of the sutures. As he sat in the reception room, the sack moved slowly at his feet. Next to him sat a sweet old lady with a cat in her arms, her eyes fixed hypnotically upon the undulating container.

Finally, no longer able to suppress her misgivings, the little lady looked up at the boa's burly owner and timorously pointed at the sack. 'What's in there?' she asked in a wee voice.

'Ten-foot boa constrictor.' A matter-of-fact reply.

'THAT'S WHAT I THOUGHT!' shrieked the old lady at the top of her voice, and desperately clutching the cat to her bosom, she threw herself against the far wall.

One episode that is particularly clear in my memory occurred when a client called to ask the fee for castrating a monkey.

Suddenly, the telephone receiver was filled with the noise of excited chattering. The monkey had picked up an upstairs extension phone and was eavesdropping on our conversation.

Like most veterinarians who treat exotic species, I have usually discouraged animals of this kind as pets, except in special circumstances. I treat these animals, but that doesn't mean I approve of them as pets for the general public. The popularity of exotic animals as pets has contributed to the loss of population in the wild, and often the owner fails to give the animal proper care and nutrition. Some of the more aggressive species are destructive, and some are dangerous.

However, during the fifties and sixties, it was perfectly legal to own many species of exotic animals as pets in Los Angeles County, and since there were very few veterinarians willing or able to treat such animals in those days, owners of exotic pets streamed to our clinic in neighbouring Ventura County.

One day a woman phoned me from Los Angeles. 'I'm told that you treat ocelots,' she said. Indeed, these attractive little spotted cats were frequent visitors to the Conejo Valley Veterinary Clinic.

'I have a chance to get a free ocelot,' she said, 'but I thought that I'd better get some advice first. What do you think of the idea?'

'I'm glad you called,' I said. 'So many people who are totally unqualified for the responsibility commit themselves to the care of an exotic pet. May I ask a few questions, please?'

'Yes, of course, and I do appreciate your time.'

'Where do you live?'

She gave me an address in a densely populated suburb in the San Fernando Valley.

'Do you have other pets?'

'Yes. We own two dogs and two domestic cats.'

'Do you have children?'

'Yes we do, ages four and six.'

'Have you ever owned an exotic pet before?'

'No. The zoo is as close as we've ever been to such an animal.'

'What is your and your husband's background and training?'

'Well, I'm a housewife. I used to be a secretary. My husband drives a truck.'

I spent the next fifteen minutes telling why I did not recommend accepting the ocelot as a pet, explaining the liability, the philosophical aspects, and the legal implications of owning such an animal. She thanked me profusely for my time.

Two months later she telephoned me again.

'I'm the lady who was offered the free ocelot and asked what you thought of the idea. You advised me not to accept it. Do you remember me?'

'Yes,' I said. 'I remember our conversation.'

'I want to thank you again for all the time you gave me, for being so honest with me, and for not letting me make a mistake.'

'You're welcome,' I replied.

'Now,' she continued, 'I want to make an appointment. We bought a mountain lion.'

Sometimes though, as any veterinarian will testify, it doesn't take an unusual creature for the problem to be out of the ordinary. I recall well one Sunday that started out quietly enough. I made an early morning call to check a horse I had seen Saturday evening. He had recovered nicely from his colic, and I left instructions to feed him. Then I went to the clinic to make my rounds. There were only two dogs and a cat in the ward. The cat's owner was waiting for me, and we let Fluffy go home with her recent spay incision already healing nicely. Both dogs were doing well: the boxer was learning to walk with a Thomas splint on his fractured foreleg: the cairn terrier had stopped itching and chewing at his paws. I drove home, relishing the thought of a peaceful day, but as I drove down the steep driveway to our home, the little house we had rented, Debby met me at the door with a wistful expression.

'Phil Garone called,' she said. 'He's on the way down to the clinic with his collie dog. She sounds pretty sick.'

The eight-year-old sable-and-white collie was depressed. 'She's been drinking a lot of water,' said Phil, 'and she won't touch food. Look how swollen her belly is.'

'When was she in heat last?' I asked.

'About five or six weeks ago.'

'Look,' I said, 'I'm going to draw a blood sample. I want to see if her kidneys are functioning properly and run a blood count. I think she may have pyometra. That's an infection of the uterus wherein the organ fills with pus, usually after a heat period. She's a good candidate for pyometra. She's eight years old and has a history, if you recall, of false pregnancies. That's a typical history preceding pyometra.'

'I don't remember,' said Phil. 'Sophie usually brings the dogs in. She's been feeling lousy, so I came this time. Everything happens at once!'

Sophie was Phil's wife, a young woman with a strikingly attractive face and jet black hair, but a rotund body. She wasn't so much obese as she was round. Like a basketball.

Lassie's blood urea nitrogen was normal. Her kidneys were functioning adequately. About half the female collies I saw were called 'Lassie' after the popular television programme. The depressed collie never moved as I drew the blood sample from the vein in her foreleg. She just sadly watched me, her chin resting on the examination table. Collies are almost always gentle, cooperative patients. Her small, sad brown eyes watched my movements.

I whistled when I saw her white cell count. Sixty thousand! It looked like a pyometra all right.

While I prepared Lassie for an exploratory surgery, Phil called his wife to tell her the bad news. By the time I was ready to make my incision, Mr Garone had arrived.

'If it *is* a pyometra, will that mean that she can never have puppies?' the globular, dark haired lady asked.

'Yes, we'll have to do a complete hysterectomy,' I explained. 'The diseased uterus is filled with pus and will be removed.'

'Oh,' said Sophie. 'I'm so sorry we never bred her. I always planned to have a litter, but I guess I waited too long.'

When I opened the abdomen, I saw something I had never seen or heard of before. Lassie had pyometra all right. Her uterus looked huge, distended and purple and filled with pus, but – she *was* pregnant. There, in that infected and abnormal uterus which would have caused Lassie's death in a few days, were living foetuses. I don't know how the five pups managed to survive the environment, but the Garones were even more mystified by how the collie got pregnant.

'We kept her locked in the yard the entire time she was in heat,' the Garones insisted. 'We *always* keep her locked in the yard! There aren't any other dogs around. We live way out in the country. You know our place!'

'Well,' I pointed out. 'Obviously a male dog did get to her!'

Lassie came through her operation nicely, and Phil brought her back twelve days later for me to remove her sutures.

'Have you heard about Sophie?' he asked.

'What about Sophie?'

Phil Garone's face broke into a broad smile. He reached into his shirt pocket and produced a cigar and stuck it into my pocket.

'I have a son! Remember I said how bad Sophie had been feeling? She felt lousy for months. Well a couple of nights

188

ago she started cramping real bad. I gave her some Pepto-Bismol, but she got worse, and I got scared and took her to the hospital emergency room in Oxnard. The doctor came out and said, 'Mister Garone, your wife is having a baby!'

I said, 'What? She isn't even pregnant! We've been trying to have a baby for six years.'

'The doctor said, "She is very pregnant, but she won't be much longer. She's having a baby, right now"!'

Phil continued to beam at me.

'You mean to tell me that your wife has been pregnant nine months and neither of you knew it?'

'Right!' Phil asserted joyously. 'You know, Sophie's kind of chunky, so we never noticed. Anyway, we have a baby boy – and you know what? That's better than having puppies!'

It's true that the life of a medical practitioner – MD or veterinarian – is busy, hectic even. If it's not emergency surgery on a Sunday, then it's something else. For example, I recall the fall that the rains came early. By December, which is right in the middle of calving season, the grass was lush and green and the pastures water-logged. I was in the midst of my rounds on a frantically busy Saturday when my office called. There was a cow down on the Lang Ranch.

When I arrived at the ranch, I went through the gate I had been instructed to and drove along the slippery road until I saw three riders ahead, waiting for me. As I neared them, my vehicle mired down in the mud.

'The ground's too soft for you to go any further, Doc!' I gnashed my teeth at the obvious pronouncement. 'The cow's about a mile up this draw. You take this horse and one of us will take you up to her, and the other two of us will get your truck out of the mud.'

Curses! Why did this have to happen on a busy day? I was irritated and annoyed. I have had to make a number of calls on horseback in my time, but this call would destroy my schedule, even if the riders were able to get my truck free. However, there was nothing I could do about it.

The cow had recently calved, and I guessed that I was going to find a calving complication, probably an injury to the obturator nerve in the pelvis, resulting in temporary paralysis of the hind limbs. I loaded my pockets and the saddle bags with everything I thought I'd need and, following the riders, proceeded uphill, still seething internally when I thought about how many visits I had to make and the people and animals waiting for me.

It was a glorious December day. The ground was moist, the grass fragrant and green. We don't have a real winter, so it was, in reality, early spring. White clouds drifted lazily in the blue sky. A meadowlark sang. The big, stout quarter horse gelding I rode walked rapidly, his head bobbing energetically. The sun warmed us. It was midday. A red-tailed hawk wheeled and shrilled above me. I stopped scowling and relaxed.

We crossed a fresh-running stream. Cows with new little calves were scattered through the pasture. I could see some of the white baby faces hidden in the brush up on the hillsides. Another meadowlark sang. I smiled. The horse climbed a rocky slope. I patted his neck. 'Good boy,' I told him. By the time we reached the cow, a white-faced Hereford with a white-faced black calf at her side, I was basking in the peace and beauty of my surroundings. This really was more pleasant than driving down the freeway to the San Fernando Valley, where several horses were awaiting me.

I examined the cow. I had guessed wrong. 'This is grass tetany,' I said. The lush new growth had caused her paralysis by causing a mineral imbalance. 'I brought the wrong drugs. I'll have to ride back to my truck to get what I need.' That meant another three miles of riding; one down to the truck, another back to the cow, and third down to the truck, again.

Why did I feel so good? I should have been furious, with the cow, with the mud, and with myself for guessing the wrong diagnosis.

A couple of hours later, I finally arrived at the San

Fernando Valley stable.

'I'm sorry I'm late,' I apologized. 'I got stuck in the mud.'

'Then how come you look so happy?' the client asked.

Chapter 31

Pierre Esponde is a Basque. He is a butcher, and he also owns a few horses. I recognized his loud and enthusiastic voice immediately over the telephone. 'Allo, Doctor? This is Pierre. I read in the newspaper about theese anthrax outbreak in Agoura. You know, the cows what die from the anthrax? Should I worry about my horses?'

Anthrax has been one of the most dreaded livestock diseases from time immemorial. It was Louis Pasteur who first developed an effective vaccine against it. All mammals are susceptible to anthrax, including man, and the disease occurs all over the world. The bacillus that causes anthrax forms spores that seem to survive forever in the soil, so once an area has had the disease, that area is permanently charted as an anthrax district. We have many such designated 'anthrax pastures' on the ranchlands in our part of California.

I have never seen a live cow with anthrax. In every case I have experienced, the animal was found suddenly dead, even when it looked perfectly normal the preceding day. That is how fast anthrax can kill ruminants. In other species, however, such as humans and in swine, anthrax can display a more chronic course.

I told Pierre that horses could contract the disease, but that I had never seen an equine case. Horses could be vaccinated, but nobody seemed to do it. All of the local cattle were vaccinated annually, but what had happened this year was that, due to drought, the cattle had grazed the grass down to the ground where the spores are, very early, before most of the ranchers had vaccinated. Hence we had an outbreak of anthrax, and everybody had rushed to vaccinate as soon as the word got around.

In any case, Pierre's horses were several miles away from the involved pastures, so I reassured him.

'Okay, Doc,' he bellowed. 'Whatever you say ees okay weeth me. 'Ey, Doc. What *ees* thees anthrax, anyway? I don't hear of eet before.'

When we studied this dread disease in veterinary school we had to learn the other names by which it is known around the world. Thus, anthrax in German is *milzbrand* and in French it is *charbon*.

'Well,' I said, 'you were raised in cattle country in the Pyrenees, so you are probably familiar with the disease as *charbon*.'

'Ooooh!' gasped Pierre over the telephone. Then, in a horror-struck voice, he loudly whispered, '*Charbon*! *Charbon*!'

Pierre certainly had heard of anthrax, and the way he said *charbon* made my skin crawl. Pierre was a butcher, and in the old days, one of the ways that humans contracted anthrax was by handling infected meat.

Several days later, Jungleland brought us a dead mountain lion, requesting a post-mortem examination. The animal had looked completely normal the preceding evening, and had eaten. This morning it had been found dead in its cage. Suspecting foul play, the owners wanted to know the cause of death.

Bob and I had hired a veterinary pathologist, Dr Gordon MacMillan, to help us out part-time. Because of his special training, he immediately assumed the responsibility for most post-mortem examinations in our practice, although his regular duties included the routine treatments of everyday veterinary practice. Gordon worked for us two days a week to supplement his income as a pathologist in a government laboratory.

While Bob saw small-animal clients, I went out into the country to see the large animals. I returned at noon and found Gordon busily dissecting the mountain lion's body.

'Find anything?' I asked.

'Very unusual,' Gordon replied, 'I'm certain that this was some sort of septicaemia. See the echymotic and petechial haemorrhages on all mucosal surfaces? Look at the heart. See the pericardial haemorrhage? Look how swollen the spleen is. What's interesting is the throat. These pharyngeal lymph nodes are extremely abnormal, haemorrhagic and inflamed.'

A bell rang in my mind. Back in school, didn't they say that anthrax in swine is characterized by such involvement of the pharynx?

'Gordon,' I said.

'Yes,' answered Gordon, busily sectioning the lymph nodes with his knife.

'Gordon, doesn't anthrax in swine show lesions like these?'

Gordon froze, looking up, startled. Then he dropped his knife and backed away from the table.

'Oh, my gosh!' he said. 'There's been anthrax in Agoura, and Jungleland picks up dead cattle to feed to the cats.'

Known anthrax carcasses are burned and buried on the spot, but perhaps someone found one of their cattle freshly dead and, not thinking of anthrax and not concerned enough to wonder what the cause of death was, simply called for the dead animal hauler.

That is exactly what had happened. We had to disinfect the hospital, Gordon was put on penicillin as a precaution, as were all of the big cats at the Jungleland zoo, and we eventually published a scientific paper describing the only recorded case of anthrax in *Felis concolor*, the American mountain lion. No doubt, however, that in the wild, this sort of thing had happened many times, but without veterinarians being present to recognize the disease.

Chapter 32

In days gone by, physicians would differentiate *diabetes mellitus*, 'sugar' diabetes, from *diabetes insipidus*, a disease in which there is no sugar in the urine, by actually tasting the patient's urine. Of course, in modern times laboratory tests have replaced this primitive and unaesthetic method.

One of the companies from which we buy vaccines always puts a few cans of frozen orange soda pop in with the shipment to keep it cold in transit. Consequently, we often have orange pop in the hospital refrigerator.

One summer we employed a veterinary student from Colorado. Among other duties, Art was assigned to run our urinalyses.

Some days we all feel particularly inspired. On such a day I transferred some orange pop from the can to a beaker. When Art came into the laboratory I handed the beaker to him and requested a urinalysis. He promptly started the test while I pretended to be busy at the microscope, awaiting his reaction.

'WOW!'

'What's the matter?' I asked.

'Look at this sugar reaction,' Art responded. 'It's loaded.'

I slapped my forehead. 'Of course! How stupid of me! 'Diabetes mellitus! It should have been obvious! Polydipsia! Polyuria! Ravenous appetite! Loss of weight! It should have been obvious, but I never thought of it! Thank goodness I had the sense to run a urinalysis!'

Art was busy with the sample. 'Let's check for ketones,' he said.

Meanwhile at his elbow, I sniffed at the beaker. 'Wow, you can smell the sugar!'

Then I touched a forefinger to the orange liquid and touched it to my tongue. I saw Art's shoulders stiffen. He appeared to concentrate his attention on the glassware, but

194

he was watching me out of the corners of his eyes.

'Wow,' I said again. 'Loaded!'

I tasted again. 'How could I have missed the diagnosis?'
Art still sat stiffly.

'Taste that, Art,' I offered.

'No thanks!' he blurted.

I lifted my eyebrows, pretending surprise. 'Hey, you're
not squeamish about tasting it, are you?' I asked.

'Damn right!' Art assured me.

'You'll have to get over that if you're going to be a
veterinarian,' I told him. 'Why, did you know that in the old
days doctors had to taste urine as a routine diagnostic test?'

'I know, I know,' he assured me. 'And mellitus means
"sweet" and insipidus means "tasteless," but no thanks! I'll
just use my little chemicals here!'

I snorted in disgust, 'Well, for heaven's sake, aren't you
delicate!' Then, immediately, I lifted the beaker and
gulped the entire thing down.

'AAAARGH!' Art gasped. 'You're insane!'

Then as I convulsed in laughter, understanding illuminated Art's face.

As has become apparent, veterinary practitioners receive
so many outlandish calls and requests in the course of their
work that nothing surprises them. After a short time in
practice they will believe anything. This makes them easy
marks for practical jokes.

One morning I arrived at the office and looked at the
schedule. Bob Kind was assigned to surgery all morning,
but there was only one brief operation scheduled for him.
He had a tomcat to neuter. So I wrote in his column in the
appointment logbook, 'Jungleland – dehorn rhinoceros.'

When Bob came in he looked at the logbook and then
mumbled to himself. Finally, he asked me, 'Is this a baby
rhinoceros or an adult I have to dehorn?'

'Bob,' I said reprovingly, 'babies don't have horns. It's
an adult – that big male they have over there.'

'Why are they dehorning it?'

'I don't know. I guess because it's so damned mean. Tried to kill a couple of the keepers.'

Bob mumbled to himself some more, looking concerned.

I offered, 'They'll probably want you to save the horn for them. I guess it will be worth a fortune down in Chinatown.'

'Yeah! Yeah!' Bob said. Then, 'Is it coming in here, or do I have to go down to Jungleland?' he asked.

'No, you'll have to do it down there. We measured the door to the clinic, and it's too narrow. The rhinoceros won't fit through the door.'

After a few minutes I could see that Bob was planning his surgical approach. 'Let's see,' he said, 'a rhino's horn is modified hair, so I assume that it does not have a bone core like a cow's horn. So, I guess if I circumscribe the base and use a Gigli wire saw. . .'

'Bob,' I said, 'it's a joke. I just wrote it down to be funny. You don't have to dehorn a rhinocerous this morning.'

Bob looked slightly crestfallen, but also somewhat relieved.

'Hey,' he said, 'in this practice *anything* is possible. I've had to repair an elephant's trunk. Why not remove a rhinoceros's horn?'

Another time I phoned the clinic on my day off and asked for Dr Kind.

'Doctah, mah boll weevils are dyin' and' ah wondah if you could hep me out?' I asked.

'I don't know anything about insect diseases,' he replied politely. 'Why don't you call the entomology department at Pierce College?'

'Ah did!' I said. 'They told me to call a vet! Ah really need hep, doctah. Ah've lost half mah weevils.'

I had his interest now. 'What is happening to them?' he asked.

'They jus' curl up and die,' I explained.

'Do you raise these boll weevils? Why are you so concerned?'

'Wel-l-l, doctah,' I drawled, 'ah'm from Texas, and the

196

weevils remind me of home. You know some folks keep ant fahms?'

'Yes.'

'Well, ah raise boll weevils, an' they're dyin'.'

Apparently deciding that he was wasting valuable time talking to a kook, Bob tried to dismiss me. 'Well, I'm sorry about your problem, but I really can't help you.'

'Wait a minute!' I interjected. 'Ah have anothah problem. Ah have to leave town for a few weeks. Could you boahd mah weevils?'

'Well,' mused Bob, 'that's kind of an unusual request. I suppose I could if you told me what to do. What do you feed them?'

'Why cotton of coahse!' I roared.

'Oh, naturally,' he sputtered hastily. Then, after a long silent interval he asked, 'Miller, are you at it again?'

Being a patient and deliberate man, Dr Kind waited for the right moment to return the favour.

An old buffalo used to graze near Thousand Oaks in a large pasture consisting of several sections of dry, hilly grassland. Driving back to the office one day from my calls, I noticed the old bull curled up close to the wire fence next to the highway. He was still there the next day, so I stopped to investigate. He was dead. It was summertime, and after a week the decomposing buffalo could be detected for a quarter of a mile in each direction from where he lay.

Bob Kind had spotted his opportunity because the next morning, to my great dismay, I read in the appointment book: 'Dr Miller, complete autopsy on dead buffalo. Send report to humane society. Information to be used in lawsuit.'

Immediately I babbled to my partner: 'Did you see that appointment book? They want me to post that buffalo that's been lying dead out in the hundred-degree heat all week!'

'Yes,' he said sympathetically, 'and they wouldn't have anybody but you. They said they want a complete examination, sections taken on all organs and tissues, and removal of the brain and spinal cord. I told them it would be very difficult to determine the cause of death because of the advanced state of decomposition.'

Looking at Bob sadly, I said with resignation, 'Well, I suppose I'd better get out there and get to work as early as possible. It's going to be a scorcher today.'

Everyone had a good laugh at my expense that day. So, you see, no request is too bizarre, too grotesque for a practitioner. He can be counted on to succumb without question to the most farfetched practical joke. It's not a character fault; it's just another of our many occupational hazards.

Chapter 33

The Circus Vargas is the only three-ring circus in the United States that still performs under canvas. There are larger circuses, but seeing these shows in a coliseum or sports arena just isn't the same as seeing a circus in a tent in the traditional way circuses were seen for centuries.

When Circus Vargas played Ventura County each spring, we would do a lot of veterinary work for them, which they would have saved up until they were in our area.

Everyone who has seen a circus is familiar with liberty acts. In a liberty act, a group of horses performs in the ring, completely at liberty and not controlled by lines, responding to the trainer's commands. The trainer usually occupies the centre of the ring.

In a three-ring circus, similar acts perform in all three rings simultaneously, the most famous act taking the centre ring. Thus Circus Vargas had three different liberty acts, each starring a team of horses of one breed.

One of the circus' liberty acts was made up of six Appaloosa stallions. The horses ranged in age from six to sixteen years. Although the act was an impressive one and the stallions performed flawlessly, off-stage they were terrors. Neither man nor beast was safe around them, and having them gelded had been contemplated for a long time. Grooms had been injured, and anytime the horses were turned loose together, they fought savagely.

Finally one of the stallions bit a chunk out of a groom's cheek, seriously mutilating the young man. That did it! The trainer decided that when the circus played Ventura County, the stallions would be castrated.

The modern Appaloosa horse is as colourfully spotted as the old-time 'appy,' which the Nez Perce Indian tribe originated. However, the modern Appaloosa usually has a lot of thoroughbred or quarter-horse blood, sometimes both. This cross-breeding has refined the modern Appaloosa's conformation and also modified the horse's temperament. The old-time 'appy' was a tough animal, physically and mentally, and these circus horses were old-time types. They were big, raw-boned, Roman-nosed, and had small, malicious eyes. They were tough.

We used a fenced pasture adjacent to the circus lot as an operating room. The first horse was led in and given a general anaesthetic. As soon as the operation was completed we left the patient lying in the grass to awaken. Then the second horse was led in, and the process was repeated. By the time I was gelding the fifth horse, the first one staggered to his feet. As I started to operate on the last stallion, the second horse also got up. As soon as the two stallions saw each other, they charged one another. Still off balance from the anaesthetic, and despite having been castrated only minutes before, they had no thought but to attack each other, and a screaming, striking, biting, stallion fight ensued.

'Get them apart!' I yelled. 'Somebody do something!'

'It's okay, Doc,' the trainer assured me. 'They do like that all the time!'

'But they've just been operated on,' I pleaded. 'They'll haemorrhage! Get them apart before they kill each other!'

While some grooms reluctantly went to find halters, the third horse lurched to his feet and, screaming defiance, drunkenly joined the fray.

By the time I had completed the last operation, four of the stallions were involved in the fight. They were separated with difficulty – and with some risk to the men who caught them.

I dispensed some bright yellow medication to spray on the incisions and left careful post-operative instructions. 'When can they go back into the act, Doc?' the trainer wanted to know.

'In a week,' I said. 'The healing will be complete enough by then that the audience won't be aware that they have recently had surgery.'

After I cleaned up my instruments, I went to the motor home that served as the circus's business office. Mr Vargas, the owner of the circus, paid me for my services, in cash as is the circus custom. Then he gave me three passes, saying, 'Here Doctor, perhaps you'd like to take your family to the show.'

I drove back to Thousand Oaks and phoned Debby from the office. 'Mark is going to see his first circus,' I told her, thinking she'd be pleased for our young son. 'We're going to Ventura tonight to see the Circus Vargas.'

'What about dinner?' my wife wanted to know.

'We'll eat at the show,' I suggested. 'Hot dogs and circus stuff. Mark will love it.'

So that evening we sat in the stands munching hot dogs and enjoying the performance. Mark kept wanting to know, 'Is that elephant your patient, Daddy? What about the lions? Do you take care of the camels? Do you take care of the bears?'

200

Halfway through the show the ringmaster called out, 'Lay-deez and Gen-tul-men – Boys and Girls – the Liberty Horses!'

Three teams of horses entered the tent, one in each ring. There in front of me were the six Appaloosas I had gelded that morning. The horses performed perfectly. Then at the end of the act, the trainer raised his whip and all six horses stood up on their hind legs, revealing the medication I had dispensed – their groins gleamed a brilliant yellow.

On another occasion Debby, Mark, and I went to another circus.

While Debby went to buy hot dogs and drinks. I took Mark to the menagerie tent to see the animals. The elephant trainer was one of my clients, and when I introduced her to my little boy, she asked if Mark would like to ride on one of the elephants in the grand entry parade. My son was speechless, but his eyes sparkled as he looked at me imploringly.

'Sure,' I said.

I returned to our seats. 'Where is Mark?' Debby asked, all maternal anxiety.

'Oh, I left him with Carol. She's an elephant trainer, and she said she'd bring him back to his seat in a little while.'

'Are you sure he'll be all right?'

'Sure!'

'He's going to miss the grand entry! Look, they're starting the parade! Mark will miss it.'

'No,' I reassured her. 'He can see it from where he is. He won't miss it.'

'Why did you leave him? He's only a little boy. He can get in trouble. He's missing the parade. He should be here with me.'

'Watch the grand entry,' I suggested as Debby craned her head, trying to catch sight of her son. 'Look at the elephants,' I urged her.

There on the head of the second elephant, holding on as tightly as he could, his face radiating excitement and happiness, was our boy!

'That's Mark!' Debby yelped, and as spectators around us looked at her, she shouted, 'That's my little boy riding the elephant!'

Judy's Elephants was the name of the world-famous elephant act. Whenever they played Los Angeles, for a circus or a television show or a motion picture, they were stabled in Goebel's barn. On one such occasion, I was called to see a sick elephant. The huge beast was losing weight, had a poor appetite, and seemed weak and listless. She was led into the concrete-rimmed training ring where I examined her.

'I'll need to take a blood sample from her ear vein,' I told the trainer, and went to my emergency bag outside the ring to get the necessary syringe, needle, and vials. As I bent over the bag, behind me I heard someone say. 'Hey! Watch her!' That was followed by a thunderous thump and a terrible crack.

The 9,000-pound creature had fainted, and as she fell, she hit her skull against the concrete ring border.

It is anguishing to see an animal this size lying helpless. The laboratory tests eventually revealed a kidney infection, but the head injury was our immediate problem. Nina, the elephant, had a brain concussion and was barely conscious. She was unable to get up. An animal this size cannot lie on its side long without internal organs failing from the pressure. Even a 1,000-pound horse will suffer irreversible organ damage if it is down too many hours, so I didn't think a 9,000-pound elephant could live long unless we could get her into an upright position. That would permit her lungs and circulatory system to function.

'She's going to die if we can't get her up,' I said.

'You want to get her up?' the trainer asked. 'We'll get her up, Doc.'

Circus people are amazingly ingenious and handy, and are masters of improvisation. Within twenty minutes they had constructed a tripod of telephone poles, and with a power hoist and thick rope slings, they had the semi-conscious elephant in an upright position.

I was able to catheterize an ear vein, and through it I poured fluids, nutrients, medication to relieve the pressure upon her injured brain, and antibiotics, which eventually relieved the kidney infection.

A few days later Nina walked up a ramp into a large trailer and was moved to Tucson for her next performance with the rest of the elephants in the act.

This time, however, Mark didn't go along for the ride.

Chapter 34

I have always had a special penchant for horse practice, but there is a physical aspect to this type of work that can be difficult at times. Horses are powerful, flighty animals, and all veterinarians who work with them suffer injuries during their career, and every once in a while a veterinarian is killed by a horse. After a particularly rough afternoon during which I encountered three uncooperative equine patients in succession, I decided to draw a cartoon depicting the anatomically ideal equine practitioner.

Starting at the top, I created a thick skull to protect the vital underlying organ. The nose was flat and boneless, making it difficult to fracture. A big mouth facilitated communication with clients and the teeth were strong, white, and prominent, providing an essential winning smile. I set this skull on a short, powerful neck.

Next followed huge shoulders supporting long, slender

arms that nearly reached the ground. These arms, terminating in long, strong, sensitive fingers, would be immensely valuable in providing extra reach for making rectal examinations, restraining tall horses, and floating teeth. The chest was barrel-shaped to accommodate substantial heart and lungs. A full abdomen made room for an extra-large stomach suitable for gorging on infrequent and irregular meals.

Finally, the legs were extremely short so that, although the entire individual was quite tall, he would have to do a minimum of stooping when working on a horse's legs and feet.

Surveying the finished drawing, I was horrified to discover that the ideal equine practitioner looked exactly like a gorilla. That's when I tore up the paper and decided never to say a word to anybody about my discovery.

Veterinarians who choose to work with horses and livestock must expect to receive minor injuries regularly. Our feet get stepped on, our toes are broken, fleeing patients cause rope burns to our hands, and we are periodically kicked, butted, gored, and bitten.

Aside from physical trauma, there are other difficulties involved in country practice. We spend a lot of time driving, and some of the roads we must negotiate are less than first class. We regularly get stuck in mud holes, and we must learn to negotiate narrow lanes, alleys, and driveways, and then back up when our work is finished.

Since veterinarians engaged in this kind of practice like animals and enjoy the out-of-doors, the above-mentioned hardships are taken in stride. However, there are two other problems that are far less bearable. One concerns meals. As a profession we eat irregularly, and we learn to eat *fast*.

Returning from an eastern veterinary meeting, I found myself aboard a jet aircraft in the company of two other veterinarians, Drs Ralph Vierheller and Phil Olsen, both California practitioners.

We took adjacent seats, with Dr Olsen occupying the aisle seat. After all three of us had finished eating dinner, the stewardess picked up our empty trays and then, tapping the miniature veterinary caduceus on Dr Olsen's lapel, she said, 'Even if you weren't wearing this, I'd know you were a veterinarian. And even without the caduceus, I know that you two are also veterinarians,' she added, nodding toward Dr Vierheller and me.

For a moment we were stunned, confused, and a little embarrassed. 'Do we have a special smell? asked Dr Vierheller. 'Or is it the intelligence shining in our faces?'

The girl laughed. 'No, it's the way you gulped your dinners. Look around this airplane. You three are the only ones who have finished eating, and you weren't even served first. You see, my father is a veterinarian. He has a mixed practice, mostly dairy cattle, in Pennsylvania. I've watched him eat like that all my life.'

Since then, during or after a hectic day, when I've caught myself frantically stowing away my nourishment, I have frequently remembered her words and forced myself to sit back, relax, and slow down.

Another problem is the weather. Let me hasten to say that in California's benign climate I have no complaints, but whenever I am out and experience cold or wind or driving rain, I think with great compassion of my colleagues world-wide who must endure these more frequently than I, plus ice and snow and bitter cold, as well. Of course, coastal California has its summer heat, but even that is negligible compared to the inferno of some of our desert areas or the stifling humidity much of the United States experiences every summer.

Having lived part of my life in the Arizona desert and part of it in Colorado where temperatures of minus 20 degrees Fahrenheit are not unusual, it always amazes me to hear native Californians complain if the mercury tops 100 or falls below 40. In fact, some Californians whine if the thermometer varies from room temperature.

One drenching rainy night during the sixties, I was called out to attend a colicky horse. Returning from the call at 3:00 a.m., my engine stalled. I coasted to a crossroad, turned off the highway, and contemplated my situation. I considered staying in the cab until daylight, but I knew Debby would worry. Therefore, I trudged onto the highway to see if I could get a lift.

The rain was falling in solid sheets. I wore a broad-brimmed Western hat which soon hung down around my ears. With an ankle-length slicker and rubber boots I looked a bit like an apparition, and the first car I flagged picked up speed as it approached me.

I realized some ingenuity was necessary, so when, after several minutes, another car approached, I shined my flashlight on my truck and then waved it back and forth. The driver, thinking I had had an accident, came to a stop. I immediately opened the car door, climbed in with my soaking clothes, closed the door, and said, 'Thanks for stopping. I'm a veterinarian on an emergency call, and my truck stalled. Will you drop me off at the first gas station in Thousand Oaks? It's five miles down the road, and there's a phone booth there. I'll telephone my partner, and he'll come rescue me.'

My host listened quietly as I finished my explanation. After a long silence, he blinked his eyes several times, stammered, and finally spoke: 'You're sitting on my S&H Green Stamps!'

Despite the difficulties we veterinarians endure, there are many youngsters eager to follow in our footsteps.

'This is my daughter's mare,' the man explained. 'My daughter's in school now. I wish she were here to see her horse wormed, but she couldn't stand to see her hurt, so she asked me to stay home from work so I could help you.'

'I understand,' I nodded sympathetically. 'The pain is intense but of short duration. In a few hours it's all over.'

He set his jaw, knowingly.

'My daughter plans to be a veterinarian,' he explained.

'Yes, I know,' I said. 'My practice is now entirely limited to adolescent girls who plan to be veterinarians.'

'She's nuts about animals,' he told me earnestly. 'Ever

206

since she was a little girl. She loves animals. And horses! She's crazy about horses, especially.'

'That's good,' I approved. 'If she's going to be a veterinarian, it is very helpful to like animals.'

He looked mildly surprised. 'That's the main thing, isn't it? She wants to take care of horses – be a veterinarian and take care of horses. I mean, the main thing is to love animals, right?'

'No,' I disagreed. 'It's important, but not the main thing. The main thing is to be able to drive backwards.'

'To drive backwards?'

'Yes! To be able to drive backwards and to enjoy driving backwards!'

'To drive backwards?'

'Yes! Like here! See your driveway? I'll have to back out up a thirty-degree slope, making two ninety-degree turns to get from your barn to the street. Everybody builds like this!'

'Oh,' he said, 'I see.' He searched my face to see if I was serious. 'We have only one acre on a hillside. We couldn't build a driveway with a turn-around.'

'I understand,' I assured him. 'My practice is now entirely limited to stables and driveways I must back uphill to get out of. I like driving backwards.'

'Anyway, Lisa loves horses. She really wants to be a vet.'

'I know, all of my clients are girls who want to be veterinarians!'

'With driveways you have to back up?' he asked incredulously.

'Yes!' I said. 'Of course there are other requisites to being a successful equine practitioner.'

'Oh, her grades are good,' he said.

'That's helpful,' I complimented him. 'And you have to be able to hold your bladder for twelve to sixteen hours.'

'Your bladder?'

'Yes! And be able to drive, eat, and write, all at once – that's important too! And it's helpful to have a high pain threshold, especially in your toes.'

'Toes?'

'Right.'

He studied me for a while, silently, trying to comprehend. 'Last time Lisa helped you with her mare. You had to put on a long glove and check the mare. Inside, you know? Lisa won't have to do that, will she? She didn't like that.'

'Of course not,' I reassured him. 'Nowadays veterinarians can limit their practice in any way they want.'

'Good,' he said, relieved. 'She already knows what she's going to do with all the money she makes. Know what she's going to buy?'

'A turn-around driveway?'

'No. Horses! She's going to buy all kinds of expensive horses.'

'That's great,' I said. 'She can afford it since she won't need plastic gloves.'

'Right!' he grinned. 'I guess we'd better get this over with, huh? I wish Lisa was here to help worm her horse!'

'I'm finished,' I said.

'Finished?'

'Yes,' I said. 'While we were talking, I wormed the horse.'

'Yes,' he brightened. 'There wasn't much to that, was there? And here I've been worrying how difficult it would be for Lisa to be a vet. That was easy!'

Veterinary medicine *is* a unique profession, a different way to make a living. No nine to five at an office desk for us. No sir! In time, we practitioners may begin to regard our work as routine, but you will rarely meet a nonveterinarian who does not regard our livelihood as exotic. Those who like animals view our work as fascinating. Those interested in medicine believe that what we do is challenging. Those who dislike both animals and medicine regard our daily tasks as, at least, repulsive, but never dull.

Any veterinarian who believes the profession is ordinary should board an airliner carrying some professional equipment and watch the reaction of the airline personnel.

I flew back east once to present a seminar on equine practice techniques to a veterinary association. The title of my presentation was 'Equine Psychology and its Application to Veterinary Practice.' During the seminar I demonstrated my method of passing a stomach tube into a horse's stomach for the administration of medication. The association had lined up a number of notoriously difficult patients for the seminar. I also planned to show some video tape films to clarify the technique.

Having once had my luggage lost in transit on one of these lecture trips, I now make it a habit to carry my equipment in a carry-on suitcase. In the suitcase were my notes, ropes, leather hobbles, a shiny brass 'stud shank' (a halter chain for restraining difficult horses), a length of plastic stomach tubing, a large syringe for administering medication through the tube, some surgical lubricating jelly, and a collection of video tape cassettes.

'What's in there?' asked the security guard as he studied the contents on the X-ray screen.

'Veterinary equipment,' I answered.

'That looks like a chain!' he exclaimed.

'Right!' I agreed. 'It's a stud shank.'

He looked at me quizzically, then suggested, 'Let's open it up.'

Peering inside the suitcase, he lifted out the leather hobbles and the chain. He looked down at the other paraphernalia, then at me appraisingly. For some ridiculous reason, I blushed and felt compelled to explain, 'Those are leather hobbles. For the feet, you know?'

He did not answer.

'For horses!'

A second security agent walked up and looked at my equipment without commenting.

'I work on horses! I'm a veterinarian! I'm on my way to give a lecture, and I use this stuff on horses.'

'Yes, sir,' said the agent, as he wearily closed my suitcase.

During the meeting I recalled the incident several times. Each time I thought about it, it seemed to get funnier. On the return trip I again had to go through an airport security checkpoint. The guard was a young woman. She studied the X-ray screen.

'I see a chain in there,' she said. 'We are required to open all luggage containing metallic objects.'

'Okay,' I smiled.

She looked at the suitcase's contents. They were the same as when I arrived, except for the addition of several large plastic syringes given to me by a drug salesman at the meeting. The syringes contained worm medicine.

'What's in here?' the young lady asked.

'Disposable syringes,' I explained.

She glanced up at me briefly.

'May I see these?' she asked, pointing at the rest of the contents.

'Sure,' I said, lifting out the hobbles and chains.

'Aah –' she started to ask something and then remained silent.

'It's restraint equipment,' I said.

Slowly her face turned red.

'Go ahead.' She waved me on abruptly.

Dr Murray Fowler of the faculty of the University of California veterinary school had an even more bizzare experience. A circus for which we provide veterinary services had a five-ton bull elephant to be castrated. Since the testes of an elephant are inside the abdomen, castration is a formidable undertaking, and the only person we knew who had successfully performed the operation was Dr Fowler. Thus, we invited him to come down to serve as chief surgeon on a team of four veterinarians assigned to the herculean task.

Dr Fowler kindly agreed to help us. He also volunteered to bring with him the anaesthetic agent and a special instrument he had designed for this kind of operation. The instrument was a steel ecraseur, about three feet long.

Wrapped and sterilized in an autoclave, it had the same general shape and weight as a submachine gun.

With the ecraseur in hand, Dr Fowler attempted to board an airliner in Sacramento, at six o'clock in the morning.

'Please unwrap the package,' directed the security guard.

'I can't,' said Dr Fowler. 'It's a sterilized surgical instrument.'

'A surgical instrument?' asked the guard picking up the 'submachine gun.'

'Yes,' replied Dr Fowler. 'I'm on my way down to southern California to do an operation. The instrument is sterilized.'

'Open it up,' demanded the guard, squinting and beckoning to a second security man.

'Please, no,' pleaded the doctor. 'I have to operate in a couple of hours. The instrument is sterilized, and I can't open it. You understand?'

'What kind of instrument is this?' asked the guard.

'It's a special instrument. It's for castrating an elephant.'

'I see! Would you mind waiting here, sir? We have some people who would like to talk to you.'

Chapter 35

Debby and I have always owned Australian shepherd dogs. The name of this breed is a misnomer that outrages Australians who have developed several outstanding breeds of herding dogs such as the kelpie and the Queensland heeler. The so-called Australian shepherd originated in California, but apparently is descended from Basque herding dogs which arrived here with shipments of sheep from Australia during the nineteenth century gold rush. The Californians, it is told, assumed that the dogs were Australian in origin, hence the name.

Whatever its origin, the Australian shepherd is an intelligent dog of striking appearance. Most of them have a blue-merle coat, and many of these have startling blue eyes, called 'glass' eyes.

Shortly after we were married and while I was still working in Arizona, we adopted Wendy, an abandoned patient with a congenital skin disease and a broken leg. Wendy was a wonderful dog, half Australian shepherd and half English shepherd, and she had inherited the extraordinary intelligence of both of those misnamed American stockdog breeds. Her aptitudes were more those of a retriever than a stockdog. She loved to swim and would go through breakers and even dive under water to fetch an object thrown for her to retrieve. Wendy brought the morning paper in for us, carried packages and mail, and if I needed a tool when I was working at the barn, Debby would simply give it to the dog and say, 'Take it to Bob!' She was a part of our life for thirteen years, and when we lost her, we lost a piece of our hearts.

Shortly after we moved to California, two of Debby's animals came to live with us. Debby called them her dowry. I have already spoken of Keno, the loud-mouthed dalmation. The other member of our growing family was China Doll, a registered quarter-horse mare Debby had acquired as a teenager. China Doll had a good ancestry. Her sire was Chub, a well-known stallion on California's Irvine Ranch. China Doll's dam was a thoroughbred mare, Will Rogers, brought up from Argentina to play polo on. Debby bought China Doll when the mare was three years old.

In 1959, when China Doll was ten years of age, Debby started barrel racing on her, and in two years of competition the dependable mare never once was out of the money, and she never knocked a barrel over in a race.

After we had been in California for a few years, Mrs Lynn's beautiful ranch was subdivided, and we bought a parcel of land on the arroyo and built our own home. The barn and corrals looked down on a stream that flowed year-round, shaded by oaks and sycamore trees.

In addition to China Doll we acquired another quarter-horse mare, and breeding them, we soon had two foals, both fillies. The next year we had another filly, and our little band of broodmares now numbered five.

By 1961, our life had changed. We had the new home, the practice was thriving, and with an associate I was no longer on emergency call every night and every weekend. It was time, Debby and I felt, to expand our family beyond the dogs and horses and cats we kept acquiring.

By December of 1962 Debby was in her tenth month of pregnancy. 'I don't understand it,' the obstetrician said. 'This baby should have come two weeks ago.'

'As long as it doesn't come on a Sunday,' I replied. Thousand Oaks did not have a hospital in 1962, and Debby was scheduled to have her baby in a Los Angeles hospital. Sunday evening traffic could be heavy going into the city.

On Thursday, December 13 I got a call to see a cow on the Morrison Ranch, home to 'Old Miracle', the cow Bob Kind saved. 'Come with me,' I told Debby. 'We're going to shake that baby loose.' We bounced through a wooded pasture to see Morrison's cow, but even though I selected a route with a maximum number of ruts, washes, and logs to bump over, the baby preferred to stay where it was.

Finally, on Sunday evening, Debby went into labour. An hour later, with her contractions coming at one-minute intervals, we were stuck in a traffic jam in the San Fernando Valley. I thought I was going to have to make the delivery myself, but reached the hospital just in time.

In a little while, I was looking at our first born, a son. For me, the exciting moments in life are small moments. Big things like my graduation and my marriage, are usually taken in stride, but I shall never forget the exultation of seeing Mark for the first time. It was the most thrilling

213

moment of my entire life.

Mark, who could *meow* like a cat and *cluck* like a chicken before he could speak a word, and eventually my daughter, Laurel, were born into an environment filled with animals of all sorts, and I cannot think of a circumstance better suited to develop a child's sense of compassion, nurturing, and responsibility.

Mark rode horseback before he learned to walk, and my happiest memories of his young childhood are of him sitting behind my saddle while I rode, his mother riding alongside on another horse, our dogs running alongside. We crossed the creek, and the splashing water would sparkle like jewels in the California sunshine. During moments like these I would think that I was the most fortunate of men to be able to work and play in the out-of-doors, always in view of undulating hillsides or craggy peaks or the reaching sea or pastoral ranchlands. My working hours were spent ministering to the needs of animals of every description and I never tired of them. At home I had my horses, my dogs, my sweet wife, and the goldenhaired little son who sat behind me, his fingers grasping the belt loops of my jeans.

Kenneth Fogelberg won't mind if I use his real name. As a fifteen-year-old boy he wanted to be a doctor, but he wasn't sure if he wanted to be an animal doctor or a people doctor. A decision was ultimately made because Dr Fogelberg is today a busy and successful Thousand Oaks physician.

Ken's mother asked if her son could watch some surgery. 'Certainly,' I said. 'I'll let you know when we have an appropriate case.'

The Fogelbergs' family physician was Joe Brisbane. Dr Brisbane had a Labrador retriever named Sam. Sam liked to eat stones, and one day I found myself, radiograph in one hand and telephone in the other, telling Joe that we were going to have to operate on his dog. Sam had swallowed one stone too many.

'When are you planning to operate?' asked Joe. 'At five-thirty this evening, as soon as I have seen my last patient,' I responded.

'May I scrub in with you on the surgery?' Dr Brisbane asked.

'I'd be honoured,' I answered, and then I added, 'I think I'll call Kenny Fogelberg. He's been wanting to see some surgery, and he'll be home from school now.'

That evening I made the incision, opening up Sam's belly. Dr Brisbane and Ken, also gloved, gowned and masked, stood alongside. Joe assisted me as I removed the stones from Sam's stomach and intestines, while Ken stood silently by, intently watching the procedure.

Ken never spoke during the operation, but his eyes, over his mask, took in every detail. I wondered what he was thinking. I wondered how this experience would affect his future, and his choice of careers.

Finally, at 8:30 p.m., we were finished. We pulled off our gowns and lowered our masks.

'Well Kenny,' said Dr Brisbane, 'what did you think of that?'

'Gosh,' said the youth, 'you fellows sure work late!'

Doctors' families are often neglected because of the long working hours. Veterinarians in country practices, almost without exception, attempt to compensate for that neglect by taking their children along with them on their rounds. So, just as soon as Mark was out of diapers he started accompanying me about the countryside on my calls, and later when his sister, Laurel, was born, she was indoctrinated the same way. My children learned to watch an abscess opened and regarded the flow of pus with aplomb. Ghastly barbed-wire wounds on horses merited only a 'Hey, how are you gonna fix that one, Dad?' The vet's kids feel important when they load syringes for Dad or offer solace to suffering animals.

When Mark was four years old, and I was working with horse, I always put him up on top of the pickup truck so he'd be out of harm's way. One day while I was treating a horse, the owner walked up to Mark safely perched on top of the truck.

'Are you going to be a vet like your Daddy when you grow up?' she asked.

'Sure,' Mark answered, 'But I'm going to work on small animals. I'm not going to get knocked around like he does.'

Chapter 36

One of the joys of large-animal practice is driving through the country-side. After a quarter of a century of making regular calls into Hidden Valley, often more than once a day, I still am thrilled each time I make the drive, at least during daylight hours when I can see the scenery. I tend to daydream when I drive, but I never do when I am called to Hidden Valley. As I drive the tortuous narrow road around lovely Lake Sherwood, I savour the spectacle of mountain peaks and sparkling water. I always look across the lake to the canyon where my home lies unseen, but comforting to me none-the-less, nestled as it is in these rugged hills. As I leave the lake behind, I enter the pastoral splendour of Hidden Valley, a place of green pastures, sleek cattle and horses, miles of white fences, and comfortable ranch homes. This is my office, my surgical suite, my practice place.

I also enjoy making calls through spectacular Las Virgines Canyon, along the scenic Pacific Coast Highway where the mountains meet the sea, into the harsh terrain of the Santa Monica Mountains, and into the lush farming country of eastern Ventura County where fine horse breeding farms are interspersed with orchards of citrus and avocado, and fields of vegetable, flowers, and grains.

Certain locations never fail to remind me of vivid cases I have seen there. At a bend in Cornell Road, I invariably remember the dystocia in an old mare that I could solve only by performing a fetotomy. The foal was already dead when I arrived, but that did not make more palatable the job of having to cut it into pieces in order to get it out. At a surburban intersection in Westlake, there is a handsome house. Whenever I pass it, I re-live the time when it was ranchland, and there, by the same gnarled oak tree, I remember holding aloft a vial of tetracycline as it flowed into the jugular vein of a heifer near death from pneumonia. I remember the telephone call I placed to the ranch foreman the next day, steeling myself for the words, 'She didn't make it, Doc!' Eighteen years later, I still feel the glow of relief and pleasure when I heard his words, 'Hey, Doc, she's up and eating this morning!'

At a bend in Cheseboro Road, in old Agoura, there is a ranch gate. Each of the hundreds of times I have passed that gate, I glance beyond to the grassy knoll in a grove of oaks, where I did the tracheostomy on Morrison's calf.

Roy Morrison had called me. 'Doctor, I've got a calf down with diphtheria, and you'd better hurry. He's not for long!' He told me that he was just a little way through the Cheseboro Road gate. Fifteen minutes later I drove through the gate. Roy looked down at a black bull calf with a white face where it was lying on the ground. I could tell by the quiet resignation in the rancher's face and the way he shook his head that I was too late. As I stopped my pickup truck next to the calf, Roy said, 'He's gone, Doctor! He died as you came through the gate!'

I looked down at the little creature. Its legs were extended, pupils fully dilated, its tongue protruded from its mouth, purple with cyanosis and oxygen starvation. As I looked, the bladder emptied, and the legs relaxed. Death had beaten me to the scene by seconds – but perhaps not. I jumped out of the truck and ran around to the calf. Putting my hand to the chest wall, I could feel the heart beating, although respiration had ceased. No time to open the back of my truck and find a scalpel. I took out my pocket knife, made a vertical slit along the underside of the neck, put the knife between my teeth, and, forming my forefingers into hooks, tore the soft tissues apart until the white segmented cartilage of the windpipe showed. I hooked my left forefinger under the windpipe, elevating it out of the incision, and then, with the pocket knife, I cut across the windpipe exposing its blue lining. The calf had an airway now, six inches below the place where its throat had swollen closed with calf diphtheria. Putting my mouth to the opening in the windpipe, I blew hard. The little chest expanded as the calf's lungs filled with air from my lungs. Again and again I blew until, miraculously, the calf coughed, spraying my face with blood and mucus. It coughed again, shook its head, and started to breathe on its own. Roy Morrison and I looked at each other in joy and disbelief. I ran to the truck, opened the back of its service unit and picked up a plastic syringe case. The pocket knife, no longer a surgical instrument, became a tool. With it, I cut off the end of the syringe case forming a plastic tube about five-eighths of an inch in diameter. I inserted this tube down into the calf's windpipe. It made a handy tracheostomy tube, and the little guy was now breathing through the hole in his neck. After an injection of intravenous penicillin for the diphtheria, I asked Roy to bring the calf in to our clinic. There we were able to perform a proper tracheostomy, and by the next day, it was obvious that the calf was going to survive.

How can you explain the joy at such an achievement? After all, the life I saved was only that of a calf, destined for eventual slaughter. Why does saving life bring such satisfaction, such exultation? Is there some deep dark motive behind my feelings? Would a psychologist say that I gloat, having triumphed over death? I know that death ultimately wins, that all of us, like the little calf, will die sooner or later. Perhaps there is a proper time for everything. Perhaps life, which I cherish, will seem less important in some distant time, but now, for me, for my patients, for that gasping little bovine, *to live* seems terribly important. All of us can look upon our handiwork with pride and satisfaction. The housewife should feel that, as she contemplates a cake coming from the oven perfectly formed. The cabinetmaker must feel that sense of pride and accomplishment as he views a finished piece of furniture, and the farmer as he surveys a crop emerging in neat rows from the soil he has harrowed and seeded. But what greater thrill than when life is in the balance of tipping the scale, cheating death, and seeing your patient survive? Those moments are *never* forgotten. That's why, after so many years, I never drive around that curve in Cheseboro Road without looking off into the pasture to the east, seeing the oak tree, and remembering how I did the trachcostomy on Morrison's calf.

The small-animal practitioner sees nearly all of his patients in the confines of his office or hospital. The country vet's practice, however, takes him everywhere, and almost every crossroad, pasture, and farmhouse is linked to memories of cases that ended in triumph, or in tragedy.

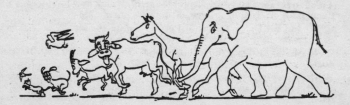

STAR BOOKS BESTSELLERS

0352315520	**TESSA BARCLAY** **Garland of War**	**£1.95**
0352317612	**The Wine Widow**	**£2.50**
0352304251	**A Sower Went Forth**	**£2.25**
0352308060	**The Stony Places**	**£2.25**
0352313331	**Harvest of Thorns**	**£2.25**
0352315857	**The Good Ground**	**£1.95**
035231687X	**Champagne Girls**	**£2.95**
0352316969	**JOANNA BARNES** **Silverwood**	**£3.25**
035231270X	**LOIS BATTLE** **War Brides**	**£2.75***
0352316640	**Southern Women**	**£2.95***

STAR Books are obtainable from many booksellers and newsagents. If you have any difficulty tick the titles you want and fill in the form below.

Name _____

Address _____

_____

Send to: Star Books Cash Sales, P.O. Box 11, Falmouth, Cornwall, TR10 9EN.

Please send a cheque or postal order to the value of the cover price plus: UK: 55p for the first book, 22p for the second book and 14p for each additional book ordered to the maximum charge of £1.75.

BFPO and EIRE: 55p for the first book, 22p for the second book, 14p per copy for the next 7 books, thereafter 8p per book.

OVERSEAS: £1.00 for the first book and 25p per copy for each additional book.

While every effort is made to keep prices low, it is sometimes necessary to increase prices at short notice. Star Books reserve the right to show new retail prices on covers which may differ from those advertised in the text or elsewhere.

*NOT FOR SALE IN CANADA

STAR BOOKS BESTSELLERS

0352316179	**MICHAEL CARSON** **The Genesis Experiement**	**£2.50**
0352317264	**ASHLEY CARTER** **A Darkling Moon**	**£2.50***
035231639X	**Embrace The Wind**	**£2.25***
0352315717	**Farewell to Blackoaks**	**£1.95***
0352316365	**Miz Lucretia of Falconhurst**	**£2.50***
0352317019	**ASHLEY CARTER &** **KYLE ONSTOTT** **Strange Harvest**	**£2.95***
0352315814	**BERNARD F. CONNERS** **Don't Embarrass The Bureau**	**£1.95***
0352314362	**Dancehall**	**£2.25***

STAR Books are obtainable from many booksellers and newsagents. If you have any difficulty tick the titles you want and fill in the form below.

Name _____

Address _____

_____

Send to: Star Books Cash Sales, P.O. Box 11, Falmouth, Cornwall, TR10 9EN.

Please send a cheque or postal order to the value of the cover price plus:
 UK: 55p for the first book, 22p for the second book and 14p for each additional book ordered to the maximum charge of £1.75.

BFPO and EIRE: 55p for the first book, 22p for the second book, 14p per copy for the next 7 books, thereafter 8p per book.

OVERSEAS: £1.00 for the first book and 25p per copy for each additional book.

While every effort is made to keep prices low, it is sometimes necessary to increase prices at short notice. Star Books reserve the right to show new retail prices on covers which may differ from those advertised in the text or elsewhere.

*NOT FOR SALE IN CANADA

STAR BOOKS BESTSELLERS

STAR BOOKS BESTSELLERS

STAR Books are obtainable from many booksellers and newsagents. If you have any difficulty tick the titles you want and fill in the form below.

Name _____

Address _____

_____

Send to: Star Books Cash Sales, P.O. Box 11, Falmouth, Cornwall, TR10 9EN.

Please send a cheque or postal order to the value of the cover price plus:
UK: 55p for the first book, 22p for the second book and 14p for each additional book ordered to the maximum charge of £1.75.

BFPO and EIRE: 55p for the first book, 22p for the second book, 14p per copy for the next 7 books, thereafter 8p per book.

OVERSEAS: £1.00 for the first book and 25p per copy for each additional book.

While every effort is made to keep prices low, it is sometimes necessary to increase prices at short notice. Star Books reserve the right to show new retail prices on covers which may differ from those advertised in the text or elsewhere.

*NOT FOR SALE IN CANADA

STAR BOOKS BESTSELLERS